Finding Love from 9 to 5

Finding Love from 9 to 5

Trade Secrets of Office Romance

Jane Merrill and David Knox

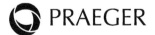 PRAEGER

AN IMPRINT OF ABC-CLIO, LLC
Santa Barbara, California • Denver, Colorado • Oxford, England

Library of Congress Cataloging-in-Publication Data

Merrill, Jane.
  Finding love from 9 to 5 : trade secrets of office romance / Jane Merrill and David Knox.
      p. cm.
  Includes bibliographical references and index.
  ISBN 978–0–313–39129–3 (hard copy: alk. paper) — ISBN 978–0–313–39130–9 (ebook)
1. Sex in the workplace. 2. Mate selection. 3. Interpersonal relations. 4. Love. I. Knox, David, 1943– II. Title. III. Title: Finding love from nine to five.
HF5549.5.S45M47 2010
646.7'7—dc22   2010027087

ISBN: 978–0–313–39129–3
EISBN: 978–0–313–39130–9

14 13 12 11 10   1 2 3 4 5

This book is also available on the World Wide Web as an eBook.
Visit www.abc-clio.com for details.

Praeger
An Imprint of ABC-CLIO, LLC

ABC-CLIO, LLC
130 Cremona Drive, P.O. Box 1911
Santa Barbara, California 93116-1911

This book is printed on acid-free paper ∞

Manufactured in the United States of America

Contents

Acknowledgments

All books are a collaborative effort. We are indebted to Michael Wilt (senior acquisitions editor, Praeger Publishers) for his interest, support, and suggestions for this project. We also acknowledge Tracie Gardner (California) and Mark Whatley (Florida) for assisting us in collecting the data. We express appreciation to the 774 Internet respondents who completed the Office Romance Survey. Leia Cain posted the Internet survey, Beth Easterling analyzed the data, and Alora Brackett provided extensive reviews of the literature on the various aspects of office romance. To the staff in the reference department of the Westport (Connecticut) Public Library—we offer our abiding gratitude. Finally, we are appreciative of the 70 individuals who shared their office romance stories during detailed interviews. To protect their identities, we have used false first names and no last names, and altered aspects of their demographics so that they would be recognized by no one.

Jane Merrill and David Knox, Ph.D.

Preface

Who has been at work and not looked up and become mesmerized as someone new entered the room? Feelings emerged with thoughts of new possibilities—particularly when the person returned the look. And who has not found working with a colleague more enjoyable than anticipated, and started looking forward to coming to work to see/be with that person?

Romance at the office has gone from being a lightening rod for a sex scandal to a fountainhead for finding a life partner.

I (Jane, first author) have worked in journalism for years and had over 20 "office jobs." I discovered early that the social part of the job was, well, part of the job. Writers went to parties, hung out at restaurants and bars, and tended to write in the wee hours. And, as research library stacks were unlikely places for either kind of sex (the wanted or unwanted), I had no prior experience of so much as winking at anyone where I worked. One editor invited me to Southampton for a weekend and proposed I bring my friends. He gave me a layout of the second and third floors of the beach house and instructed me to fill the rest in with single people I knew.

A low point was when my boss at a PR firm kept calling me into his office and showed me brochures of country inns. I told him no when he asked for a neck massage. Shortly after, he fired me (saying I was on the phone with my boyfriend when I should have been working). This was a very big firm. In my termination discussion, the head of human resources said, "You should file a complaint. You are the third woman he has hired and fired and I suspect you turned down his advances."

The still lower point was when a CEO of a company where I consulted as a public relations person stood outside my fourth story win-
dow and begged me to let him in. Had he been a stalker I might have
phoned "911," but he was my boss. I figured he traveled a lot and was
rarely seen at the workplace, so I pretended this hadn't happened.

The second author (David) is also not unfamiliar with love in the
office, as this is where he met his now wife. He has also observed the
male–female office gaming through a sociologist's lens.

Since our experience/views are limited, we collected new Internet
survey data from 774 adults and conducted 70 interviews of those who
fell in, and some out, of love on company time. These stories reveal
how the workplace, both face-to-face and virtual, is a fertile context for
discovering a new partner and launching a romance. The workplace is
also a place relevant to meeting others . . . the flight attendant meets a
passenger, the waitress meets a customer, etc. This book is for the single
person who is on the brink of an office romance or the person who is
already involved, and wondering what's around the bend.

Who's Playing at Work?: The New Internet Survey of 774 and 70 Interviews

Everywhere under the seemingly placid surface of business, there is the
undercurrent of sex, upsetting, repelling, attracting individuals . . .
Elizabeth Gregg MacGibbon, *Manners in Business*

"I owe, I owe, it's off to work I go" is the mantra of working America,
both women and men. With over 77 million men and 67 million
women workers,[1] the workplace (job, office, place of employment)
has become the primary place where the sexes meet/interact. Almost
30 percent (29%) of the adults in the United States (potential workers)
are unmarried men; 23 percent are unmarried women.[2] This book is
the story of love at the office as revealed in an original Internet survey
of 774 respondents and 70 interviews of "office" workers who shared
their tales of love and sex, heartbreak, and exhilaration. The sociological
definition of office romance is "a relationship between two members
of the same organization that is perceived by a third party to be characterized by sexual attraction."[3] A more inclusive, lay, popular definition views the office/workplace as a context where relationships may
ignite or bloom as long as one member is employed by the organization. The other party is in the role of customer or client.

Emotional/sexual relationships at the office have become common
headlines. Bill Clinton's near impeachment with the Monica Lewinsky
debacle, John Edwards's fall from grace with a journalist, and David
Letterman's monologue confession ("I had sex with women who work

for me on this show") are precursors to today's headlines of the new office affair.

Office affairs are also a part of American television culture. Now in its sixth season (and an Emmy Award winner for best comedy), *The Office* is a "docu-reality" takeoff of today's life at the office and has featured the love, flirting, and sexual relationship between Pam and Jim over a three-year period. The twosome eventually marry after Pam breaks up with her fiancé. Their office romance culminates in their wedding (with Pam being pregnant with Jim's baby).

Mad Men, now in its fourth season (and an Emmy Award winner for best drama), is set in an advertising office on Madison Avenue during the 1960s. Affairs at the office have been a recurring theme: Roger Sterling, a partner in Sterling-Cooper, has an affair with two secretaries, one of whom ends up as his wife; Pete Campbell, an account executive, has sex with Peggy Olson (a secretary) who becomes pregnant; Peggy also has an affair with Duck Phillips, her boss. The success of *The Office* and *Mad Men* emphasizes that the office is acknowledged as a major context for emotional and sexual relationships. Indeed, Obama and his wife Michelle met "at the office." Let's examine the unique social aspects of where you work.

TEN REASONS WHY THE OFFICE IS A CONTEXT FOR LOVE AND SEX

Reasons that the office/job is a place where the sexes meet, play, and mate include:

1. Dressed Up. Before arriving for their 9-to-5 work stint, both sexes are concerned about how they present themselves. Almost 75 percent (74.2%) of our Internet respondents reported that they showered before work; over 85 percent (85.6%) reported that they wore clean clothes. Men shave and women have their hair neatly combed. They look sharp, stand tall, and are quite nicely curried. Don Draper and Peggy Olson of *Mad Men* provide the quintessential examples of "dressing up for work." Don is always Mr. Good Looks and Peggy wears the latest fashion of the day (and is seen checking her belt, how her skirt falls on her body, etc). Both present their best physical selves.

2. Coffeed Up. The workplace typically includes a coffee pot. The caffeine in coffee is a mild amphetamine. Over one-third (34%) of the workers in our Internet survey reported drinking one or more cups before or during work. No wonder there is some winking going on at the office.

3. Radar On. Since most of the 32 million single men and 26 million single women in the United States will end up in the workplace, the office is

viewed as a prime place to meet a potential partner.[4] And, yes, *both* men and women are interested in more than just sex at the office: 96 percent of *both* women and men eventually marry.[5]

In this chapter, we have blended the interviews we conducted to illustrate the data from the Internet survey. Direct quotes from our interview subjects appear in *italics*. Of her office romance, one female recalled:

I had finished college and was in my first real job. I had not met a man to marry, so I was definitely looking. The prospects were slim, since the guys in the office seemed to be either losers or married. But I liked one guy who was forever complaining about his wife. After a year of water cooler talk/getting to know each other, we definitely clicked. He left his wife, I got pregnant, we lived together, and we eventually married.

And a male said:

I was ready to get married. I was 38 and tired of screwing around. When this attractive lady joined the firm, I was smitten. We dated for a couple of years and married.

4. Nice and Easy. The office provides the ideal context to move s-l-o-w-l-y through the mating ritual. *My being self-assured in my profession gives men the message that I'm detached. So instead of the guy's feeling on the spot, as though we're at a posh restaurant in Paris or Rome and have to make an instant choice from an expensive wine list . . . in a foreign language, he feels like he's sitting at a café sipping an espresso with the delicious buttery aroma in the air and a pretty girl strolling by.*

5. Peer Modeling. Most of us are influenced by our peers. If we see our friends engaging in a behavior, it increases the chance that we will do the same. In some offices, one feels an easy drift to "join the party" and become involved in an office romance, too.

6. Antidote to Boredom. Work is work and the workday is typically boring and humdrum. Love at the office offers an adventurous/fun reason for going to work and even for being alert there. It makes the hours pass quickly. Some individuals use the workplace as a playground with love and sex on the agenda. While the formal norm is that one should work when at the office (after all, that is what one is paid to do), most find interpersonal ways to make the office tolerable/enjoyable.

7. Haven for Neglected Spouses. The office/job/workplace relationship provides an alternative to an unhappy, unfulfilling, emotionally/sexually inert relationship or marriage. The spouse of an unhappy worker may be dressed in that same pair of pajamas, scowls, criticizes, complains, and coils at the touch. The unattached office worker is dressed to kill, smiles, compliments, encourages, and is responsive to the touch. There

is little wonder why relationships ignite in a context of acceptance. The lyrics of a country Western song by Patty Lovelace capture the experience of despairing spouses who engage in an alternative: "We ain't done nothing wrong, we've just been lonely too long."

For the record, we do not condone extramarital affairs. They are often devastating for spouses, partners, and children. But affairs at the office and elsewhere do occur. About one-quarter (23.2%) of husbands and 13 percent of wives in the United States report having had sex with someone to whom they were not married.[6]

8. Something in Common. Individuals are drawn to others who share their interests and background. The office/workplace provides a common set of experiences. As part of the same workplace culture, individuals have an automatic "in" on topics such as "the boss," "policies," and "office gossip."

9. Structured Contact. The office/workplace ensures that individuals will be around each other. They are literally structured into each other's lives from nine to five. With this relentless exposure, it is likely that their paths will cross, and opportunities to interact/get to know each other will unfold.

10. Context in which to Meet One's Mate. The workplace is a prime place to meet one's spouse and pair off. *I met my husband while working in forensics. Our experience of being in love and working at the same place is that you make another world, separate from what you came in with. It's no wonder people get crazy jealous of love couples at work. We can share our problems and advise each other. When you become a couple you are in a safe, new place.*

Office romances, sex, or mating are not inevitable. One female recalled:

Office romance? Sex? I thought of office sex as a fling by definition, the sort of thing that happens when you go on a business trip and are far from home. Once I went on a trip and nobody propositioned me and I thought, "I'm losing my allure."

Work is time-consuming and, for the ambitious, career minded, there may be little free time to dabble in relationships. Aware that their single employees are busy yet interested in relationships, Hitachi Insurance Service Corporation in Tokyo, Japan, provides a dating service for its 400,000 employees (many of whom are unmarried), called "Tie the Knot." Those interested in finding a partner complete an application, and a meeting or lunch is arranged with a suitable candidate, through the "Wedding Commander."

FAMOUS "OFFICE COUPLES" AS MODELS

The fact that numerous celebrity couples have acknowledged that they met at the office increases one's awareness/sensitivity to the fact that the office is a meeting/mating ground. In addition to Barack and

Michelle Obama, famous couples who met on the job include Bill and Melinda Gates, Brad Pitt and Angelina Jolie, Tom Hanks and Rita Wilson, and Chris (*Hardball*) and Kathleen Matthews.

THE NEW INTERNET OFFICE ROMANCE SURVEY

We now turn to the Internet survey we conducted to find out what is going on in today's workplace. Seven hundred seventy-four respondents completed the Office Romance Study (see Appendix A for the survey) posted on the Internet. While these individuals were primarily undergraduates in North Carolina, Florida, and California, other adults completed the survey at Heartchoice.com (Web site of the second author).

The personal identity of the respondents is unknown: the survey was anonymous (we did not capture the e-mail or IP address, or leave "cookies" on the respondents' computer). Over three-fourths (78%) of the respondents were female; 22 percent were male. Their ages ranged from 17 to 66, with most clustering during the college years of 18 to 21. Most (47%) were employed in a service job such as sales, fast food, or retail; 9 percent worked in an academic context, 12 percent in an "office," and 4 percent in a medical context. Most (73%) regarded where they worked as a "job," not a "career," and 13 percent saw it as a place to meet a future spouse.

Office Romances: Fantasy and Reality

Although almost 80 percent (79%) knew someone at work who was involved in a romance with someone else at work; only one-fourth reported that they had personally been emotionally involved with someone that they met at work. But they had been fantasizing about a romance. Over 40 percent (43%) said that they had fantasized about having a love relationship with someone at work. This latter finding is interesting. While only one-quarter actually had an office romance, 4 in 10 fantasized about a nine-to-five love relationship. In effect, these individuals were motivated to become involved and were just looking for the right juncture to make their dreams come true.

Sex

While 41 percent of the 774 respondents said that they had fantasized about having sex with someone at work, almost one-quarter (24%) had

Table 1.1   Office Fantasy and Reality (N = 774)

	Fantasized About	Actually Experienced
Love Relationship at the Office	43%	25%
Sexual Relationship at the Office	41%	24%

actually become sexually involved with someone at work. Indeed, those who fantasized about having a sexual relationship at work were much more likely to have such a relationship than those who had not done so. Is this "Wish and your dreams come true?" Table 1 reveals the percent of employees in our Internet sample who had fantasized about love and sex and the reality of their experience.

Of sex in the office, Linda (all names have been changed) in her late thirties said:

> I slept with one then another guy at my first real job, in advertising. It didn't please me. I felt like a teenage tart. I was working 45-hour weeks in a new city—no real friends, getting certified in computers at night, and no time to begin a relationship. You could say that my co-workers were "available-available" men, plus I knew I wasn't going to stay in advertising. The attraction was skin-deep with each of them. In conquering them, I was going up the first step on a staircase to conquering the city. That was 10 years ago. Since then, I have decidedly calmed down. Now I am married and have a computer consulting business with my husband. I can't believe that person who slept around the office was me.

Over 10 percent (10.6%) of our respondents noted that they had been party to oral sex on the job. Penny, 28, who manages a large optometry office, said:

> The encounters I have had at conferences are like fast food; they don't satisfy for long. They have involved nothing beyond oral sex and the anticipation—will I meet somebody in Miami? They keep me perked up about going to this kind of event, which is otherwise dull. I also make friends with guys I've slept with, which works for me.

Kissing

Almost 30 percent (28.6%) reported that they had kissed a person at work. Indeed, kissing was the most frequent physical behavior reported by those who moved from thinking about a romance to making something happen.

Rank of Person Employee Had Sex With

Almost 80 percent (79%) had sex with a peer or co-worker, 11 percent with a boss/supervisor/someone above them. Said teacher Hal: *We were both conscious of Denise's higher salary, but for me the stumbling block was "My god, this woman could fire me!"* Eight percent of our Internet respondents reported an office romance with someone of a lower rank.

Already Involved with Someone Outside the Office

Almost 20 percent (18%) of the Internet respondents reported that they were already involved with someone else when they became attracted to someone at work. Lucy taught art classes to children out of a big historic home in a one-horse town in Delaware, where she lived with her grandparents. She had been seeing the banker her grandmother favored: *"Granted he was a catch, but I felt no passion with him."* After a year of dating, she thought that if he placed a small box under the Christmas tree, she would be fooling both of them to accept. So, Lucy pre-empted a declaration by saying that she needed to "see other people."

He was taken aback, probably because for most of the year our town is a spot on the road, and the only single men are the barflies. But I was determined to give romance a chance. It occurred to me that every time I went to the mega-hardware store, my head would turn looking at some cute guy. The store is 18 miles away but I took a part-time job as a cashier. I met my husband Carson there. He is a charter boat operator who was working there in the winter in the power tool department.

Telling Others About an Office Romance

About 30 percent (28%) reported that they told someone else about their office romance. Everybody starts out not talking, then a co-worker inquires. A response of "Who, me?" seems silly, so information such as "We've gone out a few times" is disclosed.

Similarly, people are told by omission: Marc, a young editor, was full of praise for the boss's secretary—she was beautiful, smart, and a terrific girl—until they began seeing each other. Then his poker face gave him away when anyone else mentioned her. When one guy said that he would like to "do" the secretary, Marc was furious.

Sexual Harassment

About 20 percent (19%) reported that they had been physically touched at work in a way that made them uncomfortable. A higher percentage (30%) said that a person at work had said something sexual to them that made them uncomfortable (only 3% filed a formal complaint of sexual harassment).

Duration of the Office Romance

Most (18%) of the office romances lasted less than six months, 5 percent six months to a year, 5 percent between one and two years, and 2 percent five years and continuing. The remaining respondents said that they had not been involved in an office romance, so the question did not apply.

After the Office Romance Ends

Of the workplace romances that had ended, almost three-quarters (73%) ended positively: over half (54%) remained friends; 13 percent still saw each other, 5 percent married, and 1 percent lived together. Seven percent said that, compared to other relationships, the office relationship was more difficult to conclude, and 8 percent looked back on the office romance with regret. One woman said:

> If things don't work out, so much contact is unnatural. You forget and forgive but you can't get the other person off your radar. He or she circles back; you might forget yourself and resume the affair.

A slightly lower percentage recommended being open (23%) to an office romance as compared to those who recommended against it (25%). Indeed, over one-third (36.6%) agreed that they would recommend avoiding involvement in an office romance.

Losing One's Job

Less than 2 percent (1.7%) ended up losing their job at the place where they had the office romance.

Summary of Internet Survey

The picture that emerges from the Internet Office Romance Survey is that 4 in 10 of those at work fantasize about having an emotional or sexual relationship with someone in the office/workplace, and one-quarter have actually done so (with an emotional or sexual relationship). This percent is considerably lower than the almost 60 percent (59%) of employees (1050) in Vault.com's Office Romance Survey in 2010, who reported their involvement in an office romance.[7] Since our respondents were primarily young college students, we are not surprised at the higher percentage of office romances revealed in the Vault survey. To provide a more comprehensive and detailed look at office romances, we interviewed 70 older adults with experience in office romance. Details of these interviews follow.

THE INTERVIEWS

[These interviews were conducted by the first author, Jane Merrill—she has written what follows. (See Appendix B for the questions which formed the basis for her interviews.) Like researcher Deborah Tannen, her interviews were "focused conversations," where she asked the individuals about an aspect of office romance and let them talk.]

Like most women who have had a career and children, I have always had an ambivalent relationship to the workplace. I love to work. But I love to work the way I love to dance—a process and rhythm that feels right to me and favors my abilities. Because I adore the idea of a mom-and-pop business, or collaborating with a dear friend or loved one, I enjoyed conducting the interviews—talking to people about the intersection of work and love. I also enjoyed pushing aside the stereotypical responses to questions about romance in the office, and garnering what people really experienced and felt shy disclosing. Office romance was an ideal topic: it is about secret desire, secret seduction, and secret friendships in the workplace that become sexual.

Conducting the interviews I saw the office romance as an act of rebellion/detachment from the monetary goals. The people who meet and date where they work are challenging the conventional, Puritanical thinking about office romance, and those who fall in love and choose to pair up as work partners are engaged in a makeover of some of their own expectations about being a couple. How do they cope with the overlap? This became a key question in the interviews.

A focus of the interviews was to identify the potential for romance in the office in various workplace contexts. So I asked people in different professions, "What is the dating and mating scene in your profession?" I queried people employed in corporations, law firms, dental/medical offices, Wall Street/financial offices, restaurants, publishing and the media, the military, and schools and universities. I also interviewed people with an at-home business, vendors, freelancers, and part-timers who might meet someone in the course of their work. I conversed with the corporate person who had hooked up with sub-contractors (such as someone from an ad or PR agency) and the waitress who had hooked up with the restaurant manager . . . *Are there some businesses that are more conducive to finding love than others?* This was a top question for me, as it would be for a reader/dreamer of love between 9 and 5.

Initially, I conducted 70 interviews—most with women and including 20 couples—with people who had experience flirting, dating, and mating the opposite sex where they worked. Thirty of these interviews were face-to-face and 10 were on the phone. Thirty respondents preferred to share their thoughts and stories through e-mail. The age of the people I interviewed ranged from 23 to 65. Almost all were employed, and at different levels of jobs. Nearly all were college educated.

Typically, people said that they had no experience with the topic of "office romance." However, then they paused, and recollected that "there was somebody" they had dated, or flirted with extensively, who happened to work where they worked. The goal of the interviews was to get a snapshot of the workplace—what's going on in terms of sex, dating, and romance there—as a place to connect with someone special for a meaningful relationship.

To most of the people interviewed, what came to mind was extramarital activity, but they also knew of cases of people meeting spouses at work, and sometimes provided the contact to the couples (20 people) who were interviewed at length.

A woman who had had multiple jobs, from teenage through adulthood, was sure to have encountered a swaggering seducer or a Pan making conquests in the vineyard. These stories were repetitive. More interesting was how the interview subjects who were over 40 assumed that "male predators" was old-style behavior. They had a sanitized view, whereas the women in their twenties were thoroughly familiar with jerk bosses ("le plus ça change"). From feeling a shiver of desire to being infatuated to having a tryst, people spoke of a lot of sex in the workplace. These interviews revealed that the office is still a scene of seduction and amorality. The hallmark of office romances is secrecy— hiding a steamy, short or loving, long relationship between two single people, or, at the other end of the spectrum, between two people where one or both are cheating on a marriage or serious relationship. What seems very passé is that a female felt grateful to the big boss for favoring her with his approaches—the type of thing that abounds in the television series *Mad Men* or Harlequin novels.

I also heard success stories of people who had found love in the workplace and went on to combine love and work. These couples spoke of the pressures they felt as they tried to meet the emotional and practical needs of work, and love and family. They did not speak of male-female power issues; rather they pointed at the continuing need to balance being two vulnerable people in a work partnership with having the intimate current of love and sex between them. They spoke consistently of getting to know each other well, needing space, the efficiency of the arrangement of partnering work, how their relationship evolved through some conflicts, and tolerance. They reported that other people thought that they must tire of working together, but that while dealing with the bumps in the road (not balking) is fundamental, boredom was not a problem. *You're always strangers to some degree with another person,* said one of the husbands I interviewed. *You have to be civil with someone else. You can't change them. My wife is iffy in the morning. That would be true even if it were a traditional marriage, where she was dead to the world in bed and I went off on the commuter train. Instead that's something about her that factors into our work. Before eleven, I leave her be.* There is almost a level of formality as the couples who work together talk about each other.

Four of the couples were recent (within 10 years) immigrants. These couples saw their whole lives as a partnership, but viewed working together as a stepping stone to working separately. One example was a woman who was cleaning houses until her husband could build up his stonemasonry business; she could then start an import-export clothing business. Each of the four couples who chose to work together saw their situation as a temporary expediency, and did not expect it to last a generation (as did the owners of yesteryear's Chinese laundries). That was one successful model; however, new immigrants who work together want more individual satisfaction in their vocations.

Men tended to have gender specific attitudes, and reported that women are hyper-vigilant about sexual harassment. Women reported that men prowl for sex at work or in business relations. In fact, the couples who met in the workplace described a progress of their love, where hot sex and becoming special friends were intertwined. The man admiring a woman's legs, "tush," or breasts as she came into the conference room was the same man who was looking for a close person in his life.

Aside from reaffirming that the workplace is a hotbed for love and sex, the interviews revealed that no one thing is going on at the office.

Workers have all the options open to them, from clandestine sex in the supply room, to finding/marrying a mate, to no activity whatsoever. The fact that a man and woman must be more forthright than they ordinarily do about their intentions when they become serious did not seem to hold any couple back from marriage. Finally, the small sample of couples that do business together view themselves as fortunate and advantaged—an elite.

I also interviewed experts in the field of office romance—specialists whom corporations hire to alert their managers and employees to the need for caution. Dr. Marie McIntyre, a work psychologist in Georgia, is one such expert.[8] She emphasized that one can never foresee what is around the bend in an office romance. She told the story of a couple who met when working in the same department of a company. They found each other attractive, but did not pursue the attraction until the woman got a job in a different department. At that point, they had no role conflicts with each other at work, so they felt free to start seeing each other. But lo and behold, six months into the relationship, the man was promoted and became the woman's boss! So they had to sort out how they would manage that situation. They tried to end it, but the attraction was just too strong. They finally gave in and maintained a strict "no personal relationship at work" rule until one of them found a job elsewhere. Their Pas de deux goes to show that you cannot always control your circumstances.

2

Eleven Types of Office Loves

Between two evils, I always pick the one I never tried before.

Mae West

Women now compose half of the workforce in America. Many are breadwinners and many are ambitious. Feminists of an earlier generation who boldly wanted to be called Ms. instead of Mrs. or Miss projected that women would be compassionate bosses, and that innovative employment patterns, such as job sharing and workplaces with daycares, would flourish. The changes have come slowly and the scene is complex, as love and distaff life have always been.

The various office romances described by those whom we interviewed included the couple who fell in love on company time, lived together, and married; the one-sided infatuation; the office fling, where one partner was married; the office romance that went nowhere; the computer affair from the home office; an affair with the boss; and flirting with someone in the next cubicle or on the same shift with no particular goal other than to make the day pass more quickly.

Thus, the types of office romance run the gamut; however, all share one characteristic. They are all in contrast to the no-nonsense, business, make a buck culture-office romances are about play. O. Fred Donaldson states in his book, *Playing by Heart*, that "play is an act of insurrection in a dehumanized world."[1] Whether a means of passing time, telling jokes, or even cat-and-mouse and office wolf or cougar behavior, office romance occurs in the realm of play until/unless otherwise declared.

The corporate view of flirting, dating, and mating is rarely one of fear ... yes, love that flares to passion can disrupt, but repressing the attraction between men and women is not the typical response of corporate America today. To the contrary, co-opting people's private lives tacitly allows them to frolic a little to release tension in their long, intense hours at work. Some institutions even encourage love relationships on the job—parallel to serving them nice lunches or providing services as one firm does of manicurist and shoe repair. If two valued employees fall in love with each other, and both have good jobs they enjoy, the corporation wins by having two stable employees; finding two jobs elsewhere may become problematic for the couple.

Women have cleared away much of the brush of oppression. What remains? Mutual attractions that can bloom as consensual love affairs. In a study of 218 business school graduates, 30 percent admitted that they had been intimately involved with someone working in the same firm, and almost 80 percent (77%) reported that they knew of at least one intimate workplace relationship.[2] In our Office Romance Survey, one-fourth of the respondents reported emotional and sexual involvement with someone at work, and 80 percent knew of others involved in relationships at work.

While dalliance in the workplace has led to professional disaster, power struggles, and gossip, such dire consequences are not typical. What is more frequent and more important about office romance is the unequaled platform that the workplace offers for getting to know potential partners and selecting mates.

An understanding of the various types of office romances provides the basis for deciding whether one wants to play, find a mate, or both.

PLATONIC (ATTRACTION WITHOUT ACTION)

The platonic office love is management's dream scenario. Workers excel out of love for a superior, or a wish to impress a co-worker, or simply from the exuberance whipped up by feelings of intoxication around the partner. The paradigm is Money Penny and James Bond—the secretary skips to work and he reaps the benefit in her high level of performance.

Emily is a precocious 28-year-old stage manager for Broadway shows. She hardly leaves the theater, sometimes even sleeping on a cot there, while creating a show. When interviewed, she counted on her fingers the four directors she had fallen in love with. *And I don't mean a little crush*, said Emily. *I mean a raging, adoring, heartache and the disruption of my life when the show is over. Hanging on his every word, and creating a show that makes us all proud. . . . But put the two of us on a desert island and I'd never have my way with him.*

PRACTICE (GAINING MORE SOPHISTICATION AND EXPERIENCE)

In the classic dance movie *Silk Stockings*, Cyd Charisse played a beautiful Communist agent sent to Paris to round up a wayward Russian composer who has forgotten his Soviet roots and is selling out to Hollywood. Hitherto a no-nonsense political servant of the state, she is seduced by the city, and learns to be feminine, to like personal luxury, and to swoon for a mentor in romance, Fred Astaire. "What's a woman without love—a pleasure unemployed," he sings.

It is also classic for young people to learn some interpersonal dance steps on their first jobs, to explore their sexual values, and to observe behavior of co-workers whom they may imitate or drop, from how to dress to drinking a chic martini. Six seasons of *Sex in the City* and *The Office* put an accent on office romance as practice.

What are workers learning as they practice in the office context with regard to love? One lesson is the degree to which others find them attractive and the honing of their relationship skills. Said Carl, 50, who is a scientist in a pharmaceutical company:

> After my divorce I didn't know whether women would find me at all attractive. After 25 years of marriage to a woman who left me, I had reasonable doubts. I could pick up women in a bar or date one after the other via the Internet but I didn't want that. I wanted to be liked, and thought of as being okay as a person, and desirable as a physical specimen as well. I don't wear a suit to work, so I bought a new wardrobe of dress shirts and got rid of the trousers that had shrunk up over my ankles. Where I'd been aloof, I began to joke and have fun. As a scientist, I observed that the women were lighting up more than when I'd brought in a Christmas fruit cake. It helped my self-esteem to feel the reciprocal attraction months before I actually asked a psychiatrist who was in administration—Danny, my future wife, for a date.

FLIRTING TO MAKE THE WORKPLACE ENJOYABLE

Flirting is fun. Flirting is an attitude of saying "I like you" and drawing the other person out. Rosalind, a Columbia College senior in the midst of her second part-time publishing job, gave her enthusiastic point of view:

> You know the other person is in a duet with you—you're not hanging out there with your interest alone. The workplace mood is carefree and you can't invest too much; the flirting adds an extra bit of tension to a conversation without having to be on the way to anything.

Said Tasha, 24, a lab technician:

> My new resolve is to flirt with anybody, even the 80-year-old man who delivers from the medical supplier, but not to date unless it's forever. Somehow when I have my eye on a guy I look forward to getting to work. Working in a lab can be a pretty boring place to be, and that feeling of being attracted and expressing it obliquely puts a spring in your step.

TAKING A CHANCE ON LOVE

Some individuals at the office/workplace become relationship magnets, and the flirting does not stop there. A 2010 study of 5,231 employees by CareerBuilder.com (CareerBuilder.com is the nation's largest online job site) identified top locations for office romances to start: 12 percent reported running into each other randomly outside work, while other contexts included happy hour, lunch, and working late at the office.[3]

Marsha described the major theme of office romance in her life (she is 26):

> Since my first job, I have always had the spirit of a hopeless romantic, and would look for my prey, observing my male co-workers carefully. If they had a sense of humor, that was, like, my blood type and I knew that would be my object of pursuit. Nothing was really serious though, until I went to school and started my internship at a family aid center.
>
> I was 23 and I know for a fact that I fell in love with Thomas at first sight. I remember it was my first day at the internship. In walked an average-height, husky man with the brightest and biggest smile I've ever seen. Months passed until one day, my supervisor, who happened to be friends with Thomas, told me the words I wanted to hear, "Thomas likes you," followed by the words "but he has the reputation of being a player." Naturally all I heard was that he liked me, and, from there on, it was Flirting 101.
>
> There was tension, primarily because we saw each other at work, but for days at a time we didn't see each other except at work. I didn't know about his family, his friends, or his life outside the Center. We got into a huge fight and didn't speak for months; however, he was always there at the Center, so it wasn't like a usual breakup. Then my supervisor invited me to her wedding. I knew Thomas would be there, so I dressed for the occasion in a red dress and silver strappy heels. At the wedding he approached me and asked me to dance. We danced that evening, and in the middle of a slow number, he whispered in my ear that he had always cared for me . . . and that he was having a baby.
>
> A baby?
>
> It was an accident. Don't be mad!

Oh, I was definitely mad. I didn't want to take away from the wedding by making a scene, but I did walk out and cried. I couldn't believe it. Seeing him at the Center, I imagined that his love life was in abeyance, as mine was. After the wedding, I said my goodbyes, and I think that's when I made the scene. My friend pulled me away and we drove off. Thomas texted me and phoned that evening, eventually asking to come over to my apartment so we could talk. Talking led to kissing, among other things. And once again I thought I was in love. However, the next day, when I watched him with the kids and the other staff, he looked weaker and smaller. It was as though he had lost his charisma for me. He had minimized our relationship when he got a girl pregnant.

I'm a hopeless romantic. The one thing I know about dating people at work is the idea that "You think you know who you're dating, so it makes it safe" is false. When you meet someone at a bar, you have no clue who that person is: he could be a criminal, for all you know. Online dating: You set up a date and the guy ends up being 10 years older and 50 pounds heavier than he appeared to be in his picture. Friends set you up with the outcasts they rejected but didn't have the heart to stop talking to. At work, you have the illusion that you see the whole person, but in fact you are seeing only one facet of him or her. So, don't assume you know that person—you have only seen them in one context. Make sure you meet his or her friends and family soon if you are serious about the person. He or she could turn out to be someone completely different away from work. I met my current boyfriend at the grocery store—I had seen him day after day, too!

USING ROMANCE/SEX TO GET AHEAD OR TO GAIN FAVOR

In the Vault.Com 2010 Office Romance Study, 34 percent of the 1,050 respondents were aware of a co-worker whom they felt gained a professional advantage because of a romance with a coworker or supervisor.[4] This kind of jockeying for the spoils of work by putting out sexually is received with quiet loathing by co-workers, who often have to endure because they cannot "blow open" the situation to higher ups. Never mind that it is risky for the person whose job tenure may come to depend on repeated sexual favors.

INFATUATION

Infatuation involves emotional feelings based on limited knowledge of the total person. The person is seen only at work . . . showered and well-dressed, always polite. The co-worker may also be seen from afar: either because he or she works somewhere else in the building, or he or she is seen as "out of reach" in that one or both of the employees may be married. Regardless of the source, the crush of feelings is usually delightful.

Said Amy, a curriculum development specialist, age 35:

> I worked with the new principal one summer. One day I looked up when he complimented me . . . and kissed him on the mouth. I can't believe that I did that. He was a great principal and very handsome, but it was as if I was open to something before I had any idea. He was incredible, just said that that was nice, and never made me live it down. I suppose I was infatuated by him, but not in a way that interfered with either my job or my personal life.

FINDING A MATE

A switch flicks in most of us, men or women, when the flavor-of-the-month type of dating has zero attraction, and we pay more attention to ads for king-sized mattresses than to specials at the Olive Garden. The singles you know at work are people whom you trust at some level, have observed tacitly for some time, and with whom you share some education or interests. This is why the workplace has been described as the best place to meet your mate. Between 20 (Vault survey) and 30 (Career Builder.com survey) percent of office romances end up in marriage.[5]

Jennie, 32, dropped out of college and felt her college friends snubbed her. She worked for a glassblower and loved it, but there were no prospects, just her and her lesbian employer, as all the work was done for clients at a distance. So Jeannie quit and got a job in the cafeteria of a medical center where she liked the give-and-take with the customers. *I'm artistic in everything I do. I can't even fix eggs without trying a new technique, and I get along with nerds. I figured the medical center had a predominance of nerdy guys.* She dated an X-ray technician, an intern, and a physician's assistant and married the latter. *I now work at home in my own studio. We have boy/girl twins, and I know I wouldn't have met anybody as good as Dieter if I hadn't taken the reins of my destiny and switched to that job in the cafeteria.*

FATAL ATTRACTION

In 2007, Lisa Nowak, a female astronaut who was rejected by a male astronaut, was brought to trial for attempting to murder the woman who became the astronaut's next and more lasting girlfriend. When

Nowak's passion heated up and boiled over, she stalked her romantic rival 900 miles. She wore a disguise, including a wig, and an adult diaper so she would not have to stop to use the bathroom. She threatened her replacement in an Orlando, Florida, parking garage.

In another example of an office romance gone awry, announcer/baseball analyst Steve Phillips had an extramarital affair with a 22-year-old at the TV station. She was wild with desire but acted out in several "mad" ways, including driving up to his house and crashing into a wall. Phillips, it was said (probably his lawyer's advice), was not going to press charges ... but he caused the fatal attraction by becoming involved with an impressionable young woman and professing love to her. Foul play takes two!

THE EXCITEMENT IN BREAKING A TABOO

From the interviews, we discovered an astonishingly common scenario: men and women had sex in the office for no reason other than that it was forbidden ... it was something kinky to distract them from the humdrum of life. The women involved were liberal and experienced. The office sex was reported as a caper, with no or little affection attached. Here is an example:

> I was hired by my boyfriend at the insurance company after he was promoted. We often went into his office and closed the door; I gave him oral sex or we had a quickie, usually with me against the wall of the office. Across Madison Avenue were other offices, and I had the feeling that someone was watching us. That became like a slightly perverted pleasure. I'm pretty staid, but I had to move into fantasy time quickly to be responsive to sex that was over that fast.

A PLOY TO BE FIRED

Sometimes an employee is ready to be fired, so he or she initiates an office romance as a ploy to ensure that the firing happens. Sarah was a paralegal. Before becoming an attorney, she wanted to see the workings of a law firm. She was already assigned to a third-year associate when Nadia, another new paralegal of her same age, was hired. They became friends in and outside of work. Sarah found herself bragging to her friends about how amazing Nadia was. Nadia had her own personal trainer, her own masseur ... Nadia's father, a prominent lobbyist in D.C., gave her a Porsche for her birthday. But Nadia was always on the go, and it fell to Sarah to make up the work Nadia missed or did poorly. Sarah felt she could not complain to the attorney she worked for.

Meanwhile, just when Sarah was figuring that she would have to say something because her workload was getting impossible, a bunch of people in their division (including Nadia) went out for drinks. At the end of the evening, a partner in the firm put on Nadia's coat, brushed her neck with a kiss, and whisked her off in a taxi, making it clear to everyone that they were lovers . . . and he was married with a new second child, whom his wife had brought in to show off to her husband's work friends.

Still Sarah said nothing. Within a few weeks of the kiss on neck scene, Nadia was fired. "Thank God," she said as she left, "you can have everything I'm leaving, Sarah." "Including Paul?," said Sarah sharply, revealing for the first time that she knew the sordid goings on.

POWER TRIP

I (Jane, first author) began a plum consultant job one spring, as a public relations person two days a week for a high-tech engineering firm. The CEO hired me himself. He and I were both members of an Ivy League college club, and that seemed to be a good reference from my point of view. I was visibly pregnant when I met him, and felt safe enough with my big belly to accept his offer of driving with him in his chauffeured limousine to the plant, which was almost two hours out of New York City. But now that I was an employee, he had dibs on me. He proceeded to play on the tape deck dirty songs he had written and hired a musician to record.

Did I quit on the spot? No, I was about to become a single mother, with no husband to lend support, and the CEO was leaving for two months. So, I took a bus to the plant from then on, but stayed at the job for the spring. The CED let me have his office when he was away, and ond day I discovered in a desk drawer that my boss also had a "marriage business," where he brought women from Asia and matched them with American men. Ready now to quit, I asked him about all the applications that I found in the drawer—what was that about? "Yes, it's a small sideline where I find husbands for women I meet on my travels who are lonely. I try them out first." Here was a very successful engineer, entrepreneur, and father, who had let the power go wildly to his head.

THREE BASIC CATEGORIES OF OFFICE ROMANCE

Researcher Quinn studied office romance relationships and catego-
rized them as being of three basic types:[6]

1. Job related—The employee who romances another for advancement,
   security, power, or financial rewards
2. Ego—Excitement, ego satisfaction, adventure; sexual experiences exem-
   plify such motives
3. Love—Stable emotional relationship, companionship, marriage

Since most individuals have numerous jobs, they may have one or
more office romances, and the categories/motivations may vary. What
is important is that your counterpart has a motive similar to yours. For
example, if you are out for fun and adventure but your colleague is out
for love, romance, and marriage, being hurt is a certainty. Pick someone
who wants to play your game.

3

The Upside of Office Romances

Work is the number-one meeting ground where people find their spouses.

Janet Lever, Sociologist

Eliot is a Wall Street trader. With a commute totaling three hours a day, he kept his work and extracurricular lives very seperate. Although Eliot was not confessional, he conveyed over several years to everybody, including Katie, a secretary down the hall, that his relationship with his live-in girlfriend was a wasteland: He was staying with a depressed person out of fear that she would become suicidal if he left. Eliot made Katie laugh and she trusted him. Cues were given until one day they kissed in the supply room—too cliché! Katie returned the kiss and said she had regard for him, but frosted over after it occurred. Then, three months after the girlfriend burned out and went on to somebody else, Eliot realized that Katie was the love of his life. He moved slowly. They actually avoided seeing each other in the office, and the affection grew. They became inseparable, so that marriage was just tying a knot already manifest to everybody. You could say that Eliot was drawn to the comfort of the nearest femme, but theirs was also a love match, and one that would not have occurred without Katie's gutsy expression of her feelings. She said, *You're supposed to apply skills you've learned at work; well, it was reciprocal, as I applied my confidence and savoir at work to my love life. I knew I wanted Eliot, but not for a playmate. He interested me and complimented me, and I had plenty of opportunities at work to show him who I was and to see if we clicked.*

ADVANTAGES OF AN OFFICE ROMANCE

Eliot's story reveals one of the major advantages of an office romance. The fact that the partners see each other over a period of months and years allows them to observe the day-to-day happenings in each other's life . . . to see what challenges both are going through and how they deal with them . . . and to assess the degree to which they mesh with the person.

Another upside is the chance to get to know someone at leisure, said Holly, a marketing manager in a printing firm. *Tyrone worked on the shipping floor. It was a good job, but I saw him wearing work clothes and speaking English with an accent, and wondered if the divide between us was more us than just three floors. But because we saw each other time and again, and I found myself longing for those glances, I asked him to join me with our bag lunches on a park bench. I had another new boyfriend but it was as though Tyrone had a claim on me. He was a little older, had been in the service, knew several trades, and had a happy temperament that was a contrast to the "suits" I'd been dating. He became more interested in me too when I told him my goals. Because my parents gave me an apartment, and I wear jewelry and ballet slippers, he thought at first I was "cute but silly." It seems incredible that it was over three years before we did more than walk to a bench for lunch once or twice a week. And, even then, we didn't date; we both signed up for a course in framing. The attraction was evident and we were engaged before we got to the last class.*

In addition to having a long period of time to assess the merits of a potential partner, and a slow pace which allows for a deep friendship to develop, another upside of the office romance is that the nature of the work may allow the couple to create one or more products together.

Teresa and Rob met at a textbook company, where both worked in the art department. They started an affair while they were attending a children's book illustration conference. They decided to be roommates in a studio apartment in a new building for artists in their small city. They married and had success collaborating. They never had a fight—except over the fact that Teresa liked a brighter palette and Rob liked to fill the page. Soon, they were working on books together, and neither one could not tell who did what after the book came out. *People told us that if you work together as spouses you'll have a crack-up. It isn't true; we don't know how not to cooperate!*

Still another advantage to the office romance is that the workers may become more productive, not only enhancing their careers but benefiting the organization. Charles A Pierce, professor of psychology at

Montana State University, studied workplace romances extensively in terms of their effect on productivity. He noted that involvement in a love relationship at work is positively associated with self-appraised job performance. In addition, the more a person regarded him- or herself as being in love with a co-worker, the more likely the person is to feel motivated at work, to be involved on the job, and to be satisfied with one's job.[1] This is good news for corporations—turn love loose, and employees not only feel that they work harder but they enjoy their work more.

Increased work productivity may occur for two reasons: (1) The couple is not expending energy on the courtship hunt, as they have found each other; and (2) They are happy, which means that the workplace does not have to deal with absenteeism due to depression, overmedication, or loathing and avoiding one's job.

A HISTORICAL LOOK AT MEN AND WOMEN WORKING TOGETHER

Viewed from the vantage of the second half of the twentieth century, the idea that it's a plus and within the rules to meet and fall in love in the workplace constitutes a revolution. Looking back to the early settlers of America, preindustrialization, the genders were apt to work together, in the same space if not at the same jobs, given that each family produced and consumed as a unit. It is no rosy picture but reality that the sowing and harvesting, or barn raising, was done by a family and their neighbors, offering many opportunities for young people to fraternize during the important labors.

There are many similarities in the way in which men and women met their mates in the past up until now. Colonial parents influenced the choice of a spouse but did not arrange it. Young people who were working evaluated their peers to see who was socially acceptable by watching their etiquette. From the early settlement period through the periods of immigration and sweatshops to couples who meet in the arena of a university or the armed forces, the essential ground rules have remained the same: Take your time, be subtle as your relationship develops, and be aware that if the relationship fizzles, being around each other will be a challenge.

Cultural Ambivalence About Finding Love at the Office

There are some who warn that meeting a partner through work is not a good idea: it detracts from the focus of work, the boss may not like it, and you could lose your job. A team of researchers led by Janet Lever found that office romances most often do not become a problem for the corporation or the individual. In their survey of over 15,000 managers and supervisors, 90 percent reported that they "never or almost never" witnessed a workplace romance that became such an issue that someone from human resources had to get involved. And of those who had become involved with a co-worker, 12 percent reported that at least one had to be transferred or left the company.[2]

In one of our interviews, Pauline, a fundraiser for a national charity, married someone at work who was not exactly part of her job sphere. She said:

> My priority after I was at my job for four years changed from moving up the ladder to having a family. It was like I was a different person from the eager beaver who started there. The urge to settle down became so acute that I bought and furnished a house on my own. I was proud about being sought out and not seeking, but after several friends brutally told me I was sublimating, I cut down my hours at work and went to singles events . . . No luck. It was at work that I showed well, like some horse at a competition, so I stayed mindful of my wish to fall in love, and calculated who was available among the men who came and went throughout the day. One day we were gathered in my office to celebrate my birthday, and we got noisy, and an architect who was renovating downstairs banged with something on the ceiling. The next day I went to apologize, and instead of running back officiously to my office, I flirted like mad and he asked me out.

If you feel that seeking personal benefits like enjoyment and fulfillment should be outside work, then your workplace will stay arid in terms of romance. But if you are looking for love, and comfortable with yourself, you will be attractive to other singles poised to form a connection. Bruce, 35, who is employed at a large software company, said:

> The climate of my company was against being friends with anyone. The division boss would actually separate people who came to him with a new concept unless he had assigned them to work together. But when a new boss came, he didn't try to intimidate or exert authority, so the tables turned and it was okay to be friends. That's how my wife and I began—we spoke the same lingo and liked each other. I'd like to tell you that Janice thought I was handsome and irresistible, but I know our sex life started with the mind thing. She says that our ideas jumped the synapses and it turned her on.

4

Virtual Office: Love Online

> One good thing about the virtual office: You are guaranteed to click with whomever you interact online.
>
> Anonymous

The virtual office, where love relationships are spawned and developed, exists in a variety of contexts. Virtual office loves are rare (less than 1 percent of our Internet Office Romance Survey), but do occur. Some of these include the following situations.

TYPES OF VIRTUAL OFFICE ROMANCES

1. Two Employees/Same Company/Different Geographic Locations. Here, two employees of the same company meet one another in a webinar (a seminar conducted on the web). They see and talk to each other and are intrigued. They begin to e-mail privately and move the relationship forward, as do any couple who meet online.
2. Two Persons/Same Profession Meet Online. A psychologist at a university who needed gay respondents for a study on "Personalities of Gays and Lesbians" e-mailed psychology departments in other universities. One particular faculty member responded, was helpful, e-mails began . . . and continued. A virtual romance was kindled from the work role of the respective partners and continued online until they eventually met at a conference.
3. Online Office Worker Meets "Client," Who Becomes Lover. This person works from home and meets clients through the job. For example, a female airline agent who assists passengers to make plane reservations spent a lot of time on a complicated itinerary for a customer. The customer was most appreciative, expressed his thanks to her, and asked how long she had been in that role. She answered that it had been a couple of years,

and that it was a convenient way to work from home with her two children—she was a single mom. He asked what state she lived in, and they began to chat. They then began to talk and exchange e-mails after work hours. He flew out to see her, and romance bloomed.

This airline agent who works from home gives meaning to the phrase "work is something you do, not something you travel to." Over 17 million American workers sometimes work from their home—2.5 million do so fulltime. Known as telecommuting, e-commuting, telework, working from home, and working at home, these individuals typically spend their day on the computer.

4. Two Individuals Connected Online by Job Demands. Another example of a virtual office romance is an Australian physician who became a contributing editor for a New York magazine. He had frequent e-mail contact with an in-house editor at the magazine in New York. While getting their work done they began to flirt online, became enamored with each other, and presto—he flew to America and they married the next day in her apartment. (The relationship did not last, but that had little to do with the fact that they had met online—they did not experience enough face-to-face time in various contexts and "rushed" into getting married.)

5. Win-Win Relationship. A female acquisitions editor (who needed to find an author to write a book on a narrow specialty for her publishing firm) sent e-mails to faculty in various universities asking if they were writing any books. One faculty member responded that he did, indeed, have a book that he wished published. The book editor and author began a series of frequent e-mails that resulted in the editor visiting the faculty member's college. A love relationship ensued.

COMMON FACTORS IN VIRTUAL OFFICE ROMANCES

These virtual office romances have several elements in common: (1) all the lovers being unaware of each other until computer technology connected them; (2) the development of the relationship depending on the same technology that brought them together to sustain and escalate their relationship—e-mails, texting, etc; (3) each relationship became a "long-distance dating relationship."

COMPANY POLICY REGARDING VIRTUAL ROMANCES

Since virtual romances are not visible to one's boss, other policies and norms regarding employee behavior are assumed to be operative. If a company has a no-fraternization policy, it is assumed that this remains in effect for a virtual romance in which two employees work for the same company. Hence, the employees who first saw each other in a webinar and began e-mailing each other may be in violation of company policy which forbids a romantic relationship between employees. But since the boss can not see this behavior, the romance goes on without notice.

The scenario in which an employee gets involved with a customer (e.g., the airline agent helping with the complicated itinerary) would no doubt be frowned on by the company. But employees often meet the public and sometimes sparks fly; the company usually stays in the dark and can do little about it anyway. In the main, virtual office romances flourish outside the purview and control of the company.

VIRTUAL ROMANCES AS AN INTERNET RELATIONSHIP

Virtual office romances are Internet relationships, just as though the partners had met on Match.com. The parties do not see each other (face-to-face) on a daily basis and conduct their relationship online. Online relationships have both advantages and disadvantages of on-line relationships.

One advantage of a virtual office romance is that it is convenient. The employees can e-mail and text each other whenever the boss is not looking, so that each person may look forward to frequent messages from the inamorata. The parties can stay in constant virtual contact with each other.

Another advantage for those who work in the same firm is that they have a common basis of understanding. One couple who worked as account executives for Price Waterhouse noted that the pressure was grueling, but that each person had a mutual understanding of the pressure.

A third advantage is that because the employees are physically separated, they have the chance to miss, and develop an intense longing for each other. *When you are around each other all the time you tend to take each other for granted*, said a 32-year-old whom we interviewed about her virtual romance. *But being separated makes being together extraordinary.*

The disadvantages of a virtual romance include the potential to fall in love too quickly as a result of intense mutual disclosure. People who meet on the Internet tend to feel comfortable divulging their most intimate thoughts and experiences—something they may have difficulty doing in person. Since disclosure encourages feelings of closeness, two people who disclose at a high level find themselves drawn to each other.

Another disadvantage of a virtual romance is that it is impossible to evaluate "chemistry" through a computer screen. The employees need to meet in the flesh to determine if the "spark" they feel online continues in person. A common statement of people who spend months e-mailing each other and finally meet is, "He (or she) was nothing like what came across on e-mail. Talk about posting an old picture!"

Finally, virtual office romances are closed off; the parties do not interact in a social context of their friends and family (whose approval is usually crucial for a relationship to progress). One of our interviewees said that if she had known her virtual office honey had no social skills, her feelings would have been turned off instantly. But because the only incarnation of the man she "knew" was through the abstract Internet world, she did not have a clue about what he was really like.

VIRTUAL OFFICE ROMANCES AS A LONG-DISTANCE DATING RELATIONSHIP

Just as virtual office romances are Internet relationships, they are also typically long-distance dating relationships (LLDRs). The lovers in each of the five virtual relationships identified at the beginning of the chapter are all in a long-distance relationship. As with Internet relationships, there are both advantages and disadvantages to long-distance relationships.

The primary advantages of being in a LDDR include positive labeling ("even though we are separated, we are excited enough about each other to continue the online relationship to see where it goes"), keeping the relationship "high" since it is not dulled by constant physical togetherness, having time to devote to one's career, and having a lot of one's own personal time and space. Those who are suited for such relationships have developed their own autonomous/independent lives for the time they are apart, have a focus for their free time, such as their career and friends, have developed open communication with their beloved to talk about the difficulty of being separated, and have learned to trust each other since they spend a lot of time apart.

The primary disadvantages of LDDRs include frustration over not being able to be with the person you love, loneliness, missing physical intimacy, and spending inordinate money on phone calls or travel. In one study of the difficulty of long-distance dating relationships,[1] the researchers found that being separated was associated with stress, depression, relationship unhappiness, and breaking up. This is the sort of slackening of connection that "Fergie" the Duchess of York said had caused her and Prince Andrew to fall out of love, where they were for practical purposes in different companies—she in Buckingham Palace and he at sea in the British Navy. In another study that focused on infidelity, the researcher concluded that lovers in long-distance relationships were no more likely to break up because of infidelity than were partners who lived in the same town. The researcher noted that the quality of the relationship and the personality of the individuals (not compulsive) counted for more in maintaining fidelity than distance.[2]

The virtual office romance couple who want to maintain their relationship and not let the distance break them up can take the following steps:

1. Maintain daily contact. In a study on LDDRs, more than three-fourths (77%) reported talking with each other by phone several times each week (22% daily), and more than half (53%) e-mailed the other several times each week (18% daily). Some couples maintained daily contact by Web cams.[3] One respondent reported: *We get to see each other every night, in real time, using our Web cams. It has been a big help in keeping us connected. And, if we need to talk about an important issue, we can do it face to face without worrying about time or money.*

2. Enjoy/use the time when apart. While separated, it is important to stay busy with one's job/career, friends, exercise, and personal projects. Doing so will make the time pass faster.

3. Avoid conflictual phone conversations. Talking on the phone should involve the typical sharing of events. When the need to discuss a difficult topic arises, the phone is not the best place for such a discussion. Rather, it may be wiser to wait and have the discussion face to face. If you decide to settle a disagreement over the phone, stick to it until you have a solution acceptable to both of you.

4. Stay monogamous. Agreeing to be exclusive is crucial to maintaining a long-distance relationship. This translates into not being open to entanglement with others while you are apart. Individuals who say, "Let's date others to see if we are really meant to be together" often discover that they are capable of being attracted to and becoming involved with numerous "others." Such other involvements usually predict the end of the LDDR. One researcher studied 69 individuals who were involved in LDDRs and found that "moral commitment" predicted the survival of the relationships.[4] Individuals committed to maintaining their relationships were often succeeded in doing so.

5. Resolve distance problem early. Virtual office romance couples might resolve as best and as quickly as they can the desideratum of living in

the same town. Research on long-distance relationships confirms the obvious—couples who are uncertain about ever living in the same city as their online partner are more distressed, are less satisfied, and rate their communication as less effective than do couples who feel more certain about ending up in the same town.[5]

6. Other strategies. Researchers at the University of Pittsburgh revealed that partners who were separated from each other reported preserving, smelling, and wearing the clothes of a sexual partner. Over half the men and almost 90 percent of the women had deliberately smelled their absent partner's top or shirt to feel a sense of closeness.[6] A woman who was separated from her partner in the military wore his "dog" tags.

Virtual office romances come as a fringe benefit of being employed. Without warning, individuals can meet in a webinar, online, or on the phone as part of their work roles. The relationships soon take on the same characteristics of both Internet and long-distance dating relationships. These are typically out of reach of the corporate office and go virtually unnoticed; however, they may flourish.

5

Office Romance Etiquette

> Your workplace isn't that different from a party scenario. Sure, it lacks an open bar and a karaoke machine, but many of the same rules apply.
> Anthony Balderrama, CareerBuilder.com

Since the workplace is where employees meet, flirt, and explore their relationship face to face, it requires mainstream etiquette—everything you know about being civil and attentive to other people's feelings applies. According to a computer software marketing consultant with 35 years of experience, there has been a major change has occured in how companies train their personnel, in regard to the standards of human interaction, and the social side of collegial relationships that they want to see maintained in the workplace. "There used to be meetings designed to build comfortable relationships with co-workers, identify sexual harassment issues, and initiate welcome wagon-type discussion groups to inform new employees. Now it's sink or swim. You have to catch on from your co-workers and come with your P's and Q's firmly in place."[1] Various lessons that employees must learn quickly include:

FLIRTING

Flirting is rampant in the workplace. In an online survey of office romances, two-thirds of the 31,207 respondents reported that "there's a lot of flirting going on" in their current work environment.[2] Our recommendation to employees is to avoid flirting if your relationship is directed toward only one person and to never let your chats by the coffeemaker give a "we're exclusive" signal. Let the third party who approaches feel welcome.

BREAK TIME/LUNCH

Just as you are professional to include everyone in the office, the same goes for the 15 minutes in the break room. You are an employee paid to give the company store its due time. Remember that lunch may be a break from the work harness, but you must keep account of the time you spend at lunch. And if you are on a lunch date with a fellow employee, give yourselves time to end it gracefully. It's unpleasant to have to dash back to the office. Try to re-enter the workplace with dignity—not like two culprits.

COMPLIMENTS

Keep your compliments in the range of dress or job performance, not physical qualities. Even in a marriage, a woman would rather hear "You look beautiful tonight" than "You have a great ass."

INITIATING INTERACTION

Be polite and ask first . . . Ask before you suggest the merest sign of informality—"Mind if I lunch here?"

JOKES

Err on the side of caution when it comes to sharing funny stuff you see on the Internet. What would be funny off the premises may seem tactless at the office. Also, maintain your professionalism. With co-workers, this generally means no gender jokes (references to PMS, prostate problems, and so forth), and no use of trivializing words or expressions like "attaboy" or "You go, girl."

PHOTOS

If you go on a business trip together, do not post photos of it on Facebook, the office bulletin board, or "out of sight" at the edge of your computer screen.

TOUCHING

Do not depart from the helpful rule of no touching except from the elbow to the hands—what's called the "guiding touch." If you are seeing each other, viz., have attained the stage of physical fondness, keep your relationship private. This means no looks of longing, no bedroom eyes, and no touching. Even if you are sleeping together, these "love signs" can make you look like a jerk at the office.

In a study of sexual behavior at work, a team of researchers identified two types of sexual behavior—ambient sexual behavior (ASB), which involves sexual jokes, language, and materials; and direct sexual behavior (DSB), which involves direct sexual comments and advances. Of 238 employees, a majority of respondents (58%) reported experiencing at least one of these sexual behaviors in the past two years at work. Almost half (46%) of the men who experienced sexual behavior at work evaluated it positively, in contrast to 10 percent of women.[3]

THE OFFICE PARTY

Everyone likes the opportunity to get dressed up, have a few drinks, and twirl around the dance floor. Taking the women's perspective: A lot of men do not know if we are attached or not, and would rather err on caution's side. This is especially true if the men have heard even a breath about a woman in the office going out after hours, given that men do not like to be turned down (because they're men). A few dances and long looks can loosen the man's reserve. Naturally, if he has had several drinks and wants to get frisky, you have to save him from himself with a hasty retreat.

I (Jane—co-author) was so excited at my first office Christmas party (I was single). The Christmas party is generally a company's big annual bash, and employees are supposed to attend. If there is anybody at any level of the company who just might be your special one, this is where you can test the water. You can sparkle, it is jovial, nobody hears anything, and the mood is to have fun, not to watch what everybody else is doing. At my first party, by eleven, many women had kicked off their high heels. I stashed mine in a corner and kept dancing with every guy I knew. Then it was time to go home—I had come with a date. It took probably another hour to recover my shoes . . . or did I ever find them at all?

E-MAILS AND TEXTING

Avoid sending e-mails and texting from nine to five. E-mails can be read by your supervisor and used in litigation against you if things get nasty.

LUNCH WITH COLLEAGUES—THE BILL

When you go out to a restaurant with colleagues, make it clear that you alternate who pays, or pay for yourself. Do not let anybody, including your boss, pay for you unless it is work related.

ONE AT A TIME

It's a mistake to date two people at work at the same time. This cardinal rule holds true even if they are working out of offices in different states, or in divisions of the company whose staff do not interact.

YOUR PAST

Do not talk about previous girlfriends/boyfriends. It's hard to receive that kind of information and go with it. In our heart of hearts, we all want the other person to be a virgin, maybe not to sex but definitely to love. "Dan told me I was the oldest woman he'd ever dated," said Chantal. "I kept turning it over in my mind. What did he mean? Not much of anything, but I rankled at imagining this bevy of young beauties in his past. It also made me think of him as lightweight."

SNEAK A SNUGGLE?

If it feels natural to snuggle or kiss when you're in an elevator, be sure you are between floors and nobody else is in there with you. If you want to hold hands, do it someplace else, not at the office on the sly (it's human nature to be devious about sex, but do not). Even if you are doing something co-curricular, such as playing on the company softball team, remember that all eyes are on you.

DRESS

Do not wear tight clothes; instead, choose clothes that softly cling, showing off your curves. Wear clothes appropriate to your age.

Do not look as though you are reliving your high school cheerleader days, especially when it comes to skirts.

Dress with an eye to your overall reputation, not to look sexy for "him." Dress classy and business-appropriate or appropriate for a conservative occasion if it's an office party. You can be sexy without going overboard. Reputation is important, and it can precede or follow you.

Go for the sweet detail in your attire. When dressing to be attractive/noticed in the workplace, less is more has a twist. The principle is to be toned down with one extravagant element. This always catches attention in a positive way. Look at the red-winged blackbird as an example. Undistinguished on the ground, when in flight, this bird has a very red and noticeable stripe. If a woman glitters like a Christmas tree, a man turns his attention away. His eyes are more inclined to search for the hint of beautiful breasts, hips, eyes, or legs. Likewise men are drawn by a little exaggeration better than complete subtlety. That need to zoom in when a woman is wearing plainer clothes is more exciting to a guy than the drop-dead outfit.

FOOD

Laugh if you will, but a number of men and women interviewed used food to curry interest. This went from making brownies and cookies to bringing a tasty or a simple lunch (something that smells good when it heats up, like cinnamon buns, not garlicky leftovers, please). If attraction is in the air, food makes a metaphorical connection to intimacy

PACING YOUR RELATIONSHIP

The idea is not to let the relationship freeze-frame at work. First you go on a non-date . . . e.g., you go together to the gym, or you help the person choose a new couch, or you go on a charity run together. You want to be seeing each other to some extent outside the office before you get it on in the office.

Your gifts to each other should be basic courtesies and kindness combined with a low-profile sensitivity to keeping mum (no bouquets on the desk).

If you are working on a project together, keep a yardstick between you. Limit your e-mails to each other to 10 words—"Sure, see you at 6 at Macalaster's Pub!" Do not say anything you would not say to a friend. Follow this rule and you will have a brilliant, slow-building, risk-proof future with the person you are seeing from the office.

If you are seen by your boss at a restaurant or movie, be calm—you have a right to be together. If the boss asks later whether you are seeing each other, answer "Yes." Say no more. You need not say that your relationship interferes with your work performance because it does not.

WHAT IF?

What if you feel uncomfortable with a member of the opposite sex? Married or not, be proactive. Say a stirring hello and goodbye and be on your way.

How do you behave the morning after? Some people act cool and collected, but you will need your "I'm so professional" mask firmly in place if you are a bit uncertain about the relationship. No sexy words and no sexy whispering at the office, but be sure you are going to meet someplace soon where you can scintillate, be giddy, or express how you honestly feel.

OFFICE DATING—A CAVEAT[4]

Dr. Marie McIntyre, a specialist on office romances who gives corporate talks on this subject, noted what is most ignored by employees who get involved in office romances. She said:

> One common problem is that people in the throes of an office romance tend to think they have a cloak of invisibility and that no one is noticing the change in their relationship ... which is almost never the case. So they may say or do things that are not really appropriate.
>
> Another problem is rushing into a sexual relationship too quickly. People in the throes of lust are seldom patient, so they often fall into bed without considering how this change in the relationship will play out on Monday morning. When one party realizes that this was a mistake or views it as a casual fling, and the other sees it as the beginning of a beautiful romance, the working relationship is going to be toast. And the people around them are going to be very uncomfortable for a while.
>
> Office couples need to separate their work and personal relationships just like office spouses. This is sometimes harder at the beginning of a relationship, since people who are smitten often find it hard to act "normal" around each other. They need to keep their hands to themselves and resist the urge to discuss their love life with their office buddies.
>
> When people who work in the same group decide that their dating relationship is going to continue, someone needs to tell the boss. Managers need to know about such a significant change in workplace dynamics.

And the couple also needs to describe how they will keep this relationship from affecting their work or the office.

Finally, office couples need to be sure that they never try to manipulate projects, tasks, or trips in order to maximize time together. That would be unethical.

MISUSE OF POWER: IT'S NOT JUST ABOUT MEN

Now that women have more power, its appropriate and lawful use has become an issue for women, as well as men. Northern Ireland's Protestant leader, Peter Robinson, was forced out of office by a scandal when it was revealed in 2010 that his wife Iris had had an affair with a 19-year-old lover two years before (she was 58). The scurrilous and lamentable part was that she had helped her lover secure a loan of thousands of pounds sterling that the lover used to open a café. Iris Robinson had the dual position as a representative to British parliament and to Northern Ireland's Regional Assembly in Belfast.[5]

6

Dating Up and Down the Ranks

Don't sleep with the boss
Never sleep with the boss
You'll never turn a profit and you'll take an awful loss
Don't sleep with the boss

Susan Werner

Dating someone in a different rank was the theme of the 2009 romantic comedy *The Proposal*, in which Sandra Bullock plays a boss (Canadian in New York) so awful that when she exits her office, her assistant (Ryan Reynolds) e-mails the whole office that "The witch is on her broom." He is so servile that when he gets her a cinnamon latté in the morning, he orders a second cup just in case one spills on his way into the office. The script plays with this role reversal. When Bullock tells the CEO that she will not have to be deported because she's engaged to her assistant, the CEO responds, "Isn't he your secretary?" She retorts: "It wouldn't be the first time one of us fell for our secretary."

Dating someone of a different rank at the office is not unusual. Based on a sample of 5,231 workers, CareerBuilder.com's 2010 study of office romance, 30 percent of the women and 19 percent of the men reported that they had dated someone of a higher rank in their organization. By comparison, 37 percent reported having dated a co-worker at some time during their careers.[1] Our own Internet Office Romance Survey data survey revealed that 11 percent had dated a boss or someone of a higher rank.

Former U.S. Secretary of State Henry Kissinger identified power as the greatest aphrodisiac. Women are often thought to be awed by male power, while men are often thought to revel in appearing powerful to women. The evolution toward equality between the sexes is not going to alter that, although role reversals certainly seem to be more common, and the dynamic can play out differently in same-sex relationships. Navigating your relationship, when one of you has higher rank and more power is trickier by far than when two of equivalent rank make love on the boss's dime.

Contemporary novels and movies such as *The Proposal* point up that in today's workplace, men do not always have the position of power. And these novels or movies can also make it look like a lot of fun to have an office romance where you are two equal pals. In the 2009 thriller *Duplicity*, two ex-spies, played by Julia Roberts and Clive Owen, go on a corporate espionage mission for rival CEOs. As they pursue a top-secret product whose patent will bring a fortune to the agents as well as the two companies, Roberts keeps one-upping Owen, who keeps tricking her. She is a bit more eager for the big payoff than he is, and both of them are having a ball. The dark comedy is provided by the distrust the romantic pair feel about each other's scheming, every step of the way. However, by the movie's end, these attractive agents of corporate espionage are on a par, thick as thieves, and they team up for love and life.

However, perhaps a more realistic view can be found in the first two great American classic novels in which romance rears up in the workplace: *The Financier* (published in 1912) and *An American Tragedy* (published in 1925), both written by Theodore Dreiser. Both are still resonant for today's office romances. The novels' plots are based on the rise of an industrious young man who gets sexually involved with a woman he meets through work (a bank client's wife in the first novel, a subordinate at the factory in the second). The young man in *The Financier* shows genius in buying and selling stocks but gets soft in the head with regard to two women, the daughter of his mentor at the bank and the older woman, his client's wife. Dreiser's character, *The Financier's* protagonists, Frank Cowperwood, is ultimately too needy physically to keep to the austere lifestyle that it would take to achieve lasting success.

An American Tragedy was published by the time of the Great Depression (this novel was also the basis of the movie *A Place in the Sun, 1951*) and tells the story of a lowly employee in his uncle's factory. While impressing the owners by his work ethic and demeanor, Clyde dallies with the pretty seamstress. She gets pregnant and is ultimately drawn into a tragic demise.

This novel is the archetype of the top-down romance that takes a bad turn when the person with more power thinks the subordinate is standing in the way of greater success. *An American Tragedy* reveals the trajectory of two people as they trip down the wrong path. Dreiser sets the scene for tragedy even before their first embrace, noting that there was a taboo against factory girls "aspiring toward or allowing themselves to become interested in their official superiors. Religious, moral, and reserved girls didn't do it." Alas, it was too late to avert the movement of the story to a tragic finale.

OFFICE ROMANCES OF UNEQUAL RANK

According to a survey of 218 recent business school graduates, women are still perceived as entering into relationships for motives different from men, especially exploiting sexuality for gain.[2] Such a perception can make workplace relationships even more problematic for employers—why most films seem may try to avoid such problems.

As taking a different track, IBM no longer prohibits a romantic relationship between a manager and a subordinate. Rather, the corporation asks managers to step forward, make known their relationship, and ask for a transfer to another job within the company. This puts the responsibility on the manager.

In another example, an ambitious editor in a major publishing company shot her arrow at the editor in chief, and later broke up with him. She did not in the least separate love from work. And sometimes, if one of the employees is married, the romantic pair will have to live down the scandal as part of their future lives, as when Tina Brown married Harold Brown, editor of the *London Times* and her boss at the time.

In a more recent example, and one more typical of the still different reactions that the public may have to men or women in workplace relationships, *Late Show* host David Letterman was not on equal footing with the female staffers with whom he had affairs. However, Letterman's ratings and advertising appeared unmarred. By comparison, Stephanie Birkitt, his former assistant, went on paid leave (after her boyfriend tried to blackmail the famous host), and was dogged by photographers, and from now on will be known as "The Woman Dave Letterman Slept With" (something to which Monica Lewinsky can relate). As Baird observed, "Your career should never be in the hands of someone you are regularly naked with."

Another of Letterman's flames to have worked on his show, Merrill Markoe, a producer with five Emmy Awards, posted a statement about the scandal on her Web site as follows: "Okay. Here it is. My big comment on Mr. Letterman . . . It is this: As you can imagine, this has been a very emotional moment for me because Dave promised me many times that I was the only woman he would ever cheat on." According to Michelle Roehm, senior associate dean of faculty and the Board of Visitors Professor of Marketing at Wake Forest University in Winston-Salem, North Carolina, research shows that we give the benefit of the doubt to "scandalized entities"—we are more inclined to overlook their behavior—if we think it is something commonly done. Roehm calls the "show business as usual" factor.[3] Consequently, the employee does not even have the gratification of the straying person's thorough disgrace.

Then again, in the words of Stephen Crane, every sin is the result of a collaboration. An employee must summon up the maximum self-awareness and self-respect, and keep one eye open for the person who will use a higher position to throw them off-balance, or view them as ready prey. From the time we scoop ice cream or work at a summer camp we learn gradually not to fall into this kind of booby trap, whether it is velvet-lined or more obvious. Those who think they can play games with sex and sleep with the boss, or the secretary, without repercussions usually find out they are terribly wrong.

The parlous situation that Senator Max Baucus and attorney Melodee Hanes created for themselves (which came to light in late 2009) is an object lesson in how a boss-subordinate relationship can trail you. When Baucus, head of the Senate Finance Committee and one of the most powerful men in the Senate, nominated his girlfriend for the post of U.S. attorney for his home state of Montana, he neglected to mention that the two of them were bedfellows. When the story came out, Baucus's office said that the senator and Hanes began their affair in mid-2008, after the senator had separated from his wife. At the time, Hanes was employed as Baucus's state director in Montana. Baucus said that he withdrew Hanes's name from consideration for the U.S. attorney position after she moved to Washington and the pair decided to live together—presumably someone on his staff asked some questions, and gave him good advice.

Since Baucus did not have the authority to nominate anyone to the judicial post, and only recommended his girlfriend's nomination to the White House, he did not violate any rules that would cause the Senate Ethics Committee to find him culpable. Nevertheless, Hanes's legal credibility could be tainted because she was amenable to getting a leg up from her lover for career advancement. If the typical male-female fallout from the boss-subordinate affair holds true, she is the one who is more damaged, while Senator Baucus's arrogance in recommending his girlfriend for such a post is ascribed to the typical King Ape behavior. Had things gone smoothly for Hanes, it might have been worse for morale in the U.S. attorney's office; people who worked for her would have had to bear up in silence. They might suppose that undue influence placed a powerful senator's girlfriend there over other candidates.

CONSENSUAL RELATIONSHIP AGREEMENTS (THE "LOVE CONTRACT")

Whenever workplace problems exist, employment lawyers are not far behind. Some lawyers now draft agreements which office lovers may be asked to sign to protect themselves and/or the company from a sexual harassment or discrimination suit if the relationship goes sour.

The letter agreement excerpted below, written by Jeffrey M. Tanenbaum, a partner at Nixon Peabody LLP (who is widely credited with writing the first love contract), can be adapted to any type of relationship in the workplace.

This letter was sent by a top executive of a company to his subordinate (assistant vice president) with whom he was involved in an office romance:

Dear [Name of Object of Affection]:

As we discussed, I know that this may seem silly or unnecessary to you, but I really want you to give serious consideration to the matter, as it is very important to me. . . .

I very much value our relationship and I certainly view it as voluntary, consensual and welcome. And I have always felt that you feel the same. However, I know that sometimes an individual may feel compelled to engage in or continue a relationship against their will out of concern that it may affect the job or working relationships.

It is very important to me that our relationship be on an equal footing and that you be fully comfortable that our relationship is at all times fully voluntary and welcome. I want to assure you that under no circumstances will I allow our relationship or, should it happen, the end of our relationship, to impact on your job or our working relationship. Though I know you have received a copy of [our] company's sexual harassment policy, I am enclosing a copy . . . so that you can read and review it again. Once you have done so, I would greatly appreciate your signing this letter below, if you are in agreement with me.

[Add personal closing]

Very truly yours,

[Name]

I have read this letter and the accompanying sexual harassment policy and I understand and agree with what is stated in both this letter and the sexual harassment policy. My relationship with [name] has been (and is) voluntary, consensual and welcome. I also understand that I am free to end this relationship at any time and, in doing so, it will not adversely impact on my job.

[Signature of Object of Affection]

Mr. Tanenbaum has also developed a more legalistic agreement for workplace relationships that have become more problematic:

STIPULATIONS

The Parties stipulate that:

> A. *Employee 1] is presently employed by the Company in the position of [position].*
> B. *[Employee 2] is presently employed by the Company in the position of [position].*
> C. *[Employee 1] and [Employee 2] each are voluntarily engaged in a mutually consensual relationship ("Consensual Relationship") with the other.*
> D. *[Employee 1's] desire to undertake, pursue and participate in said Consensual Relationship is completely and entirely welcome, voluntary and consensual and is unrelated to the Company, [Employee 1's] professional or work-related responsibilities or duties, or [Employee 1 or 2's] respective positions in the Company or business relationship to each other. As of the date this Acknowledgment and Agreement is executed by [Employee 1] agrees that nothing in any way related to, stemming from, or arising out of his relationship with [Employee 1], has resulted in, or has caused a violation of the Company's Sexual Harassment Policy or any law or regulation.*
> E. *[Employee 2's] desire to undertake, pursue and participate in said Social Relationship is . . . entirely welcome, voluntary and consensual [etc., duplicating the entire preceding paragraph to cover the female employee]. . . .*

AGREEMENT

1. [Employee 1 and 2] have carefully reviewed the Company's Sexual Harassment Policy, a current copy of which is attached hereto. . . . understand

and agree to abide by and be bound by that Policy and any amendments or changes to that policy.

[The agreement then requires the signers to notify a supervisor or HR for the company of any violations of the sexual harassment policy or related laws, or if the relationship is "negatively affecting in any way the terms and conditions" of their employment.]

. . .

5. The Company shall immediately investigate the reported violation, suspected violation or incident and take any and all appropriate remedial action, up to and including termination, pursuant to Company policy and law. Appropriate steps will also be taken to deter any future violations or incidents.

6. Employee 1 and 2 understand and agree that conduct or speech in the workplace which is sexual or amorous may be objectionable or offensive to others. Therefore, Employee 1 and 2 agree not to engage in such conduct on Company property or when performing work-related tasks in public areas. Such prohibited conduct includes, but is not limited to, the following: touching in a sexually suggestive manner; sexually suggestive gestures; sexually suggestive speech or communications, whether oral or written; and display of sexually suggestive objects or pictures.

7. Employee 1 and 2 acknowledge and agree that each, respectively, has the right and ability to end said Consensual Relationship at any time without repercussion of any work-related nature, and without retaliation of any form by the other.

. . .

14. The Parties, having read all the foregoing, including attachments, and . . . having been notified of the right to seek the advice of counsel and having understood and agreed to the terms and conditions of the Acknowledgment and Agreement, do hereby execute said Acknowledgment and Agreement by affixing their signatures hereto.

Signed and Dated: By: [Employee 1]

Signed and Dated: By: [Employee 2]

Dated: By: [Company Representative][4]

While these agreements and contracts are not romantic (particularly the longer version), they can help protect all involved if love goes awry (and no one would deny that is possible).

Not to be totally discouraged, if you fall for your boss, sex oppression does seem to be on the wane, and men in particular seem to be learning that abusing their power with an intern at the office is not only callous, but stupid. If you fall for your single boss, if there is reciprocal love, and if the circumstances are right for a life together, you may be one of the lucky ones. With spouses aiming toward sharing and communicating in marriage today, you do not have to feel that the "boss" will have the negative habit of lording it over you outside the office!

For others, while you are figuring out whether to respond to your boss's play for you, you can watch *Mama There's a Man in My Bed*. In this French comedy, an African immigrant single mother saves the day for her tycoon boss—whose wife is unfaithful and whose next-in-command is poisoning the yogurt so that the company will have to sell out—and love blossoms. The highly intelligent and life-experienced woman will not put up with any condescension or moral slackness, and only loves the CEO when he really changes and sees her as an equal.

However, like any affair, an office romance can follow you like a bunch of tin cans on a string. Paul's second wife had been a paralegal before they married. Another attorney, whom she had chosen not to marry, was not invited but showed up at the wedding—he was a big, burly guy with a threatening presence and visibly upset. The bride's office sex followed her all the way to the altar.

I'm a night person, said Carey, *so I became an au pair and went to school at night. The unthinkable happened, and the mother I was working for died in a car crash. The husband asked me to stay on. Then he asked me to be his wife. I loved the children, naturally, and loved him. But the circumstances were all wrong. I stayed two more years, until I finished my degree, and I admit, we slept together, which he thought meant I agreed to be possessed, but once he was on his feet I left—the upstairs-downstairs pattern was too apparent and strong.*

OFFICE ROMANCES OF EQUAL RANK

In 1991, during the Persian Gulf war, when the *USS Acadia* returned stateside, 36 women (out of the 360 women in the crew) were no longer aboard due to medical transfers for pregnancy. It caused the Navy acute embarrassment when the destroyer was derisively called the "Love Boat."[5] The Navy denied that there was improper fraternization between men and women after the ship was at sea. However, in a similar case in 2009, the commanding officer was held responsible, with an admission by the Navy that fraternization occurred on the leader's watch. Commander Paul Marquis, skipper of the destroyer *James E. Williams*, and the ship's top enlisted sailor were removed and reassigned to administrative duties on shore in the wake of nine fraternization cases between senior and junior enlisted personnel on the ship.[6]

By an order enacted in November 2009, Major General Anthony A. Cucolo, who at the time had charge of U.S. troops in northern Iraq, made getting pregnant or impregnating a fellow soldier (although consensual) punishable by court-martial and jail time.[7] In making the existing policy stricter, he stressed that sex between deployed military was a problem that the Army could deal with. Because of the top-down command, the military can make decisions about behavior, i.e., regulate it to a much greater extent than, say, it can be regulated in the general public or civilian workplaces.

"The Navy was okay with our dating," said a sailor referring to her affair with her future husband. "We were sent to the same advanced training facility when we told our commanding officer that we were engaged, and we saw each other off-base there as much as we could." It is interesting that a couple can date and marry and continue their career in the Navy—if they are not markedly divided by rank. When Jane's (first author) daughter, Julia, was in Navy boot camp in the Great Lakes training facility, she found that male and female recruits were thoroughly integrated in basic training—according to Julia, none of the instructors bemoaned any loss of rigor from genders. All recruits—male or female—were on par and put through the same paces, Julia's graduation ceremony was a model of gender-integration symbolism and remarks.

When people at the same level date, a power differential does not pertain; however, employers and co-workers will still be concerned about potential problems, and gossip can be a major issue. *Suddenly everyone thought I was Mata Hari*, said the assistant director of a city aquarium. *It was either show us the ring, or break it up. I was shocked to be the subject of gossip just because I was dating one of the biologists. We didn't have a chance to let our relationship develop naturally because we were under pressure to commit to each other. At an opening for an exhibition, someone on the board of directors came up to me and said, "Oh I understand we are going to have a wedding here next." It was like having parents push you—too much for me!*

The work productivity of peers who work in a team with these individuals may also be negatively affected.[8]

WHEN BOTH FEEL THAT THEY MARRY UP

The Vows section of the *New York Times* reported on Josh Gaudet and Gita Pullapilly, a documentary filmmaking team who made *The Way We Get By*. The documentary is about the Maine Troop Greeters, several dozen elderly greeters who meet every soldier passing through the Bangor International Airport on his or her way to or from Iraq and Afghanistan with cheers.[9] When they met in December 2004, Josh, of Bradley, Maine, and Gita, the daughter of Indian immigrants of South Bend, Indiana, were a producer and reporter for competing Grand Rapids, Michigan, television stations. Josh was thinking of making documentaries, and a colleague suggested he talk to Gita, who was also seeking a change. "Mr. Gaudet was all business when he and Ms. Pullapilly first met in February 2004, asking her, 'So what do you want to do with your life?'" According to the column, they "began a fast friendship" and "talked shop constantly" until, said Josh, with each season of the TV show they liked to watch, we sat a little closer and then, one evening, Gita lay down with her legs in my lap . . . I told Gita that I wanted to date her." Josh proposed in December 2007. At an April 2009 screening, the subject of their wedding plans came up, and how they had put all of their money into the documentary. A wedding planner happened to be in the audience. She was touched by the film and got vendors to give them a pro bono wedding. The bridegroom told his wedding guests how after a recent Capitol Hill screening, he and his bride had met with Vice President Biden. "The Vice President told me that he had once met a man who shook his hand, looked at Mrs. Biden, and said 'You really married up.' Without missing a beat, Mr. Biden looked at Gita, then looked at me, grinned, and said, 'You're about to marry up, boy.'"

JEFF TANENBAUM'S DEVELOPMENT OF THE "LOVE CONTRACT"

I first wrote what has come to be known as a "love contract" over 20 years ago in response to a request from a client who was looking for additional assistance in avoiding problems from a relationship in the workplace. This client, a senior executive of a mid-size technology company, was actually concerned about his own workplace relationship with a subordinate. As he explained to me, as far as he knew the relationship was terrific, but how could he possibly know what his subordinate might really be thinking? He was concerned that she might feel compelled to be in the relationship or stay in the relationship just because of his senior position in the company. And he did not want that at all. There was no evidence whatsoever that this was the case, but he had been agonizing over this question. He had also recently read about a sexual harassment claim brought by a subordinate employee at another company after her relationship with a senior executive soured.

My first reaction was that these two people needed a relationship counselor, not a lawyer. When I suggested just this, my client was quite adamant that this was not the issue at all; instead, he was thinking beyond his own interests in the relationship. He wanted to make sure that he not only protected the interests of the love of his life (and employee), but also the interests of his company.

The company in question already had an extensive anti-sexual harassment and anti-discrimination policy and had trained all executives, managers, and supervisors, as well as rank and file employees on these subjects. In fact, I had personally conducted the executives', managers, and supervisors training sessions. The potential issues that can arise from relationships in the workplace were already addressed in the policy and in the training program. We agreed that I would give some thought as to what we could do that would be new and different to further highlight these issues, and to protect both the employer and employees.

A few days later, I came up with something I called a "Consensual Relationship Agreement." The basic terms of this letter agreement were contained in this chapter. The purpose of this letter agreement was several fold: (a) to highlight the importance of making sure that any workplace relationship remain consensual and welcome; (b) to make sure both parties to the relationship understood their rights and obligations under the company policies; and (c) to help ensure that if any problems in the relationship developed that could impact on work that the parties involved would follow the terms of the company's anti-harassment policy.

I was not sure how the employee would react to the letter agreement, but it was well received—and also received with good humor. As it turns out, this is a pretty typical reaction to the agreement. The agreement and relationship both worked out well.

I have written quite a number of these agreements in the years since and they have proven to be quite effective in avoiding problems from workplace relationships for all the parties involved. I have also found it to be an effective tool to help employers avoid a common dilemma that arises from a related type of HR policy. It is not unusual for some employers to adopt a policy prohibiting workplace relationships or a policy prohibiting workplace relationships between employees in a reporting relationship to one another. These policies are obviously an attempt to avoid some of the same problems that are addressed in a consensual relationship agreement. However, such policies are problematic. We all spend so much time at work that it is simply a fact of life that relationships will develop. It is very difficult, if not impossible, for an employer to effectively enforce such policies and no employer really wants to have to be a relationship cop. Further, any problems that arise often get exacerbated because employees are fearful that they have been in violation of a company policy prohibiting workplace relationships and thus these relationships go underground. When this happens the employees are afraid to bring problems that arise to the attention of a supervisor or HR and the problems just escalate from there. A consensual relationship agreement can be a useful alternative to these problematic policies.

Shortly after I wrote my first few consensual relationship agreements, it became clear that I also needed a different type of agreement for a different situation. My original letter agreement was written for a relationship that was healthy, happy, and in full bloom. This obviously is not always the case and sometimes relationships have already become problematic in the workplace for one or both of the individuals involved in the relationship. And sometimes it has become problematic for co-workers who may have to witness unpleasant and sometimes terribly inappropriate behavior. Co-workers also often have concerns about the potential for favoritism when an executive, manager or supervisor is engaged in a relationship.

I felt that these more immediately troublesome relationships may need a stronger response and I wrote a more rigorous form of consensual relationship agreement. The goals are the same but this more rigorous form, which is rarely greeted with humor, further highlight the potential risks that the parties involved in the relationship face and further emphasizes the parties' obligations to behave appropriately in the workplace. This book contains excerpts from such an agreement in this chapter.

In the years since, some reporters became aware of the use of consensual relationship agreements and began writing stories about them. The term "consensual relationship agreement" apparently is just not snappy enough for headlines so the agreements were quickly dubbed "love contracts." When I first saw such a headline I was not impressed. My reaction was that it was not a very good name for the agreements because, as Tina Turner would say, "What's love got to do with it?" I was not interested in trying to manage "love" in the workplace in any way. I was interested in making sure that a relationship of any sort, be it based on love, lust or simply convenience, would not become a problem in the workplace. However, the term "love contract" stuck. After early appearances in TV shows such as *Ally McBeal* and comic strips such as *Cathy*, love contracts started showing up all over the place and the term entered the popular lexicon. Now, I even find myself calling them love contracts and thinking "why the heck didn't I think of that in the first place?"[10]

7

What He Is Thinking

When you're in love, it's the most glorious two and a half days of your life.
Richard Lewis

In this chapter, we revisit the idea that men and women are, by nature and socialization, very different, and we take a look at how this impacts the way in which men view women. We also emphasize that men are biologically driven to seek sex with women and explore how this affects their thinking. We end the chapter with the various types of men who inhabit the office and the various types of women they "see" in the office.

MEN AND WOMEN ARE WOEFULLY DIFFERENT

It is a given that men are very different (in both biological and socialization backgrounds) from women. A list of some of the differences include:

- *Chromosomes:* XY for male; XX for female
- *Gonads:* testes for male; ovaries for female
- *Hormones:* greater proportion of testosterone than estrogen and progesterone in the male; greater proportion of estrogen and progesterone than testosterone in the female
- *Internal sex organs:* epididymis, vas deferens, and seminal vesicles for male; Fallopian tubes, uterus, and vagina for female
- *External genitals:* penis and scrotum for male; vulva for female

That biology (chromosomes, hormones, etc.) is an important determinant of being male or female is best illustrated by the experiment of the late John Money, psychologist and former director of the now-defunct

Gender Identity Clinic at Johns Hopkins University School of Medicine (Baltimore). He encouraged the parents of a boy (Bruce) to rear him as a girl (Brenda) because of a botched circumcision that had destroyed the infant's a penis. Dr. Money argued that gender was learned rather than innate. So, if the parents treated a child as a girl (e.g., in name, dress, toys), the child would adopt the role of a girl and then later that of a woman. The parents followed Dr. Money's advice—the child was castrated and the parents, under the direction of Dr. Money, set out to rear their biologically born son as a girl (they changed the child's name to Brenda, put ribbons and dresses on the child, etc.).

The experiment failed miserably: As an adult, he (David Reimer—his real name) reported that he had never felt comfortable in the role of a girl and that he had always thought of himself as a boy. He later married and adopted his wife's three children. David's story was chronicled in the book *As Nature Made Him: The Boy Who Was Raised as a Girl*.[1] His courageous decision to make his personal story public rendered support to the point that one's biological wiring dictates gender outcome. David Reimer noted in a television interview, "I was scammed," referring to the absurdity of "the experts" trying to rear him as a girl.

The point for office romances is that men and women are very different beings: they are structurally, physiologically, and cognitively different. And these differences have implications for what men and women want out of an office romance. In short, men may be more about the sex and women more about romance and the relationship. One aspect of these distinct motives is what men believe about women.

MEN'S BELIEFS ABOUT WOMEN

In one study, men were asked to indicate the degree to which they thought various beliefs were true about women.[2] These differences are shown in Table 7.1. We also show the degree to which women thought the beliefs were true.

Let's look more closely at the beliefs men have about women.

1. Women are after a husband. Eight in ten men in the survey believed that women, including those at the office, are focused on marriage. The truth is that both women and men want to get married: over 96 percent of U.S. adult women and men aged 75 and older have married at least once.[3]
2. Women are manipulative. Almost 60 percent of the men in the survey believed that women have a trick up their sleeve. Sometimes the male

Table 7.1   Gender Differences in Beliefs About Women (N=326)

Beliefs About Women	% Men Believing	% Women Believing
Women want marriage, not cohabitation	84.0%	68.2%
Women are manipulative	58.3%	33.3%
Women are controlling	58.2%	36.4%
Women assume that men are mind readers	55.4%	40.8%
Women are possessive	52.1%	32.9%
Women love money	16.7%	3.5%
Unmarried women aged 30 years are unhappy or depressed	16.3%	6.2%

A. McNeely, D. Knox, and M. E. Zusman, College Student Beliefs About Women: Some Gender Differences, *College Student Journal* 39 (2005):769–774. Used by permission.

view—that women want to get married and are manipulative—merge. Jack is one of the men we interviewed. He was convinced that Amy feigned pregnancy to nudge him to marry her. After they married, she suddenly announced that she was no longer pregnant. They divorced. Women today rarely resort to this devious tactic to provoke a marriage proposal, but even the looming possibility of it accounts for some of the paranoia that men may have about women.

3. Women are controlling. Equally as insidious as the belief that women are manipulative, almost 60 percent of the men in the survey believed that women are controlling. No wonder men shy away from relationships! Of course, *everyone* is controlling in the sense that everyone has an agenda and wants to influence their partner toward that agenda. Power is defined as the ability to influence the behavior of others while resisting the influence of others. "You Made Me Love You (I Didn't Wanna Do It)" is the title of a classic love song that captures an awareness that partners seek to use love to control each other. And men are particularly sensitive to women as "controllers."

4. Women assume that men are mind readers. Men feel that they are unfairly expected to know what women want. Over half (55%) reported that their previous partners expected them to know what they were thinking. "What's wrong?" asked Matt of his new office mate. "You know," she replied.

5. Women are possessive. Over half (52%) of the male respondents believed that women were overly possessive. Fred, speaking of his previous relationship, said: "She got angry when I so much as looked at another woman ... Lord help me if I get a text message from an old girlfriend."

With the exception of 60 percent agreeing that marriage is a goal, most of the women in the survey did not agree with the perceptions of the men. The women did not view themselves as manipulative, controlling, mind reading, or possessive. No wonder women feel as though men are standoffish. And no wonder men slink around the office fearing that they are marital prey for manipulative, controlling, obsessive women.

So, the workplace/office/job context is one in which the sexes are often wary of each other. Some men and women are polite to one another but feel safest when they keep their distance. But some break through their hesitancies, flirt, and make it clear that they are open for business in the romance/sex department. And men are typically the aggressors (particularly where sex is the goal).

THE URGE TO MERGE—MEN ARE BIOLOGICALLY DRIVEN TO SEEK WOMEN

In spite of their rhetoric that women are controlling, possessive, manipulative females whose sole goal is to get a guy to marry them, men can't help themselves when confronted with an attractive woman. Their urge to merge is biologically driven by high levels of androgen and other sex hormones to which the male brain was exposed during prenatal development.[4] Hence, men in the office will predictably have their radar on for women. Although a man may only look, and never flirt or respond to an overture, his radar is on.

The evolutionary purpose of this drive is to ensure that the species is continued. Suppose all males were completely indifferent to all females. There would be no sexual behavior, no pregnancies, no babies. The human species would literally die off. But nature has devised a way to ensure that sexual behavior occurs: it has wired men to seek young women with whom to procreate, since young women are more fertile and produce more healthy offspring than older women. Of course, men can "override" their biology and keep their sexual aggression in check. But the sexual energy is there and drives the behavior of men to initiate contact with the female.

THE MINDS OF MEN: TYPES OF MEN AT THE OFFICE

While most men have considerable testosterone, they vary in their level of aggressiveness and in how they view the women in the office. Indeed, in any workplace, job, or office there are different men with different mind sets toward the women at work. These various types include the following:

1. Mr. Ego. This is the womanizer, the good-looking guy with wavy black hair and probably a hard body who thinks women can't resist him. He wants to play and have sex, and he is clear about his intentions. Getting women into bed is an ego experience for him. In a study of 218 business school graduates, almost half (47%) said that men who have affairs with women in the office are primarily motivated by their ego.[5]

2. Mr. Love. At the other end of the spectrum are the men who are marriage minded. Mr. Love is single and looking for love. In the above-mentioned study of business school graduates, 41 percent said that men who have affairs with women in the office are primarily motivated by love. His relationship with lady love begins with a polite smile, hanging around the copy machine longer than necessary, and asking the woman for lunch. He hopes this could be the start of something big.

   Indeed, this is the fellow for whom the single marriage minded woman has been waiting. He is not only single but he is developmentally ready to settle down. He is in his early to mid-thirties, his buddies are already married, his career is established, and he's ready to mate/have children. He scans the office/workplace for a potential life partner and is ready when you are.

3. Recently Separated. This man is still reeling from fights with his ex-wife and hassles about getting to see his kids. He is consumed with minimizing the damage to his children, and fears that a "new" woman will complicate matters. Even though he is not on the market for a permanent relationship, this man will respond gratefully to polite hellos . . . and he'll be back in the water sooner than he knows.

4. Divorced. The divorced fellow has found his footing. Although still recovering economically, he knows when he will see his children again. He misses the comforts of marriage and scans the office to see if anyone there is a possibility. He may be on Match.com or eHarmony at night. He is fearful, but ripe for the picking.

5. Happily Married and Not Available. While it is assumed that all men have cheated or will cheat, the data suggest otherwise. Not only are three-quarters of husbands faithful throughout their life, those who have strayed are faithful most of the time. On any given year, 95 percent of husbands are faithful.[6] Leave the happily married guys alone.

6. Unhappily Married and Available. Married men are vulnerable to an affair if they are unhappy at home.[7] While being unhappy in one's marriage does not induce an affair, it makes a person vulnerable. Especially if the unhappy relationship with his wife includes less frequent sex (it often does) or not the kind he wants (oral/anal/frequent/hyperathletic). Suddenly the girls at the office look extra attractive, and flirting comes

easily. Sooner rather than later, a woman who flirts back finds the relationship escalating rapidly. Mr. Married may break loose and you could be the next wife. But be careful. He needs a couple of years between the end of his current marriage and a new one with you . . . so slow this train down. This relationship typically will go nowhere if you are his first outing since marriage. Again, be careful.

Married men who have had a number of previous affairs are on the prowl. These men have lost most of the barriers to having an affair and are as aggressive as some single men. Avoid them—they will use you and then move on to the next girl.

Impulsive, married men represent another category of men. They view girls on the job as sexual targets. They are up for the next time someone suggests going out for drinks, watching porn at work, you name it. They are ready for a good time, and women at the office are on the menu.

7. Living Together and Not Available. Similar to the married guy, the cohabitant or man who is engaged/has a girlfriend is typically off the list. Unless the relationship with the fiancée goes sour, this person will be the good office worker who is not interested in (and resistant to) playing, romance, or sex. The cohabitant men who are interested in an office romance have the same characteristics as those who are married and open for an affair—they are unhappy in their relationship, have a history of cheating, and are impulsive; moreover, it's clear that a woman who sidles up to them is looking for trouble. And this takes us to our next set of postulates.

HOW MEN CATEGORIZE WOMEN AT THE OFFICE

Men think of women as belonging to different categories, which include the following:

1. Miss Love. In the study of 218 business school graduates, over half (52%) said that women who have office affairs are primarily motivated by their love.[8] This woman has it together—a job, an apartment, solid family relationships. But time is passing, and she'd like to find a husband and have children. She is available. But sex won't be free. She will be slow to have sex and only if she perceives that the relationship is going somewhere. She is ready to jump aboard the romance/sex train but only if it is going into the marital station.

2. Miss Adventure. This woman is ready to play. Twenty-one percent of the women involved in office affairs are viewed as in it for adventure.[9] She is not interested in love or marriage, but in a high-pitched sexual adventure with one or more guys in the office. She enjoys sex, and younger guys may be on the menu (Ms. Cougar?). She doesn't care who knows.

Men in the office are ambivalent about her. They are attracted to her sexually, but fearful that she may be too callous, treat them as boy toys, and take complete control. This is unnerving and dispiriting. They also dislike the idea that she doesn't fancy them individually but just wants "a" man.

3. Miss Promotion. This is the woman who uses sex to get ahead. Since men are more often in positions of power, she uses her sexuality to elicit favors from the boss. As noted earlier, 17 percent of women who have affairs in the office are perceived (by the graduate business school respondents) as doing so for reasons of advancement (only about 1% of men are).[10] Some of this may be inadvertent. The woman may become involved with a man of a higher status only to discover that there are other benefits involved.

4. Miss Relationship Upgrade. This is the married gal (or maybe she has a boyfriend) who is looking for a relationship upgrade. She is pretty and sexy, and she knows it. She is used to turning men's heads. Her goal is to use sex to get a guy to sign on with her. This won't cause problems with her husband or boyfriend—she's already checked out emotionally.

5. Miss Afraid. This woman is unsettled. She doesn't like her job, her living situation is not working out, and the last two boyfriends cheated on her. She hates office politics, sees the office girls being hit on, and deflects (or doesn't "see") innuendos that come her way. She feels any office romance will have a bad ending.

6. Mrs. Married but Flirty. This is the pretty woman who is dazzling to behold at. She talks of her husband and kids and says she is happy. Maybe she is. In the meantime, she can be a flirt. And maybe that's as far as it goes.

7. Mrs. Married and Off Limits. This is the woman who is clearly committed to her marriage and shows zero interest during any interaction with any man for an office romance. It isn't going to happen.

8. Miss Hot Number in a White Dress. This woman is, in her own fashion, dressed to kill, but dresses down. Colors are muted, but everything matches and is name brand. She flirts under the radar and is coy. Eventually she agrees to a date and is a firecracker in bed.

9. "Sexutary." One of our interviews included a boss man in a small real estate firm who referred to his secretary as a sexutary. In addition to doing his bidding in reference to the job, she occasionally provides him sexual favors. The exchange was time off and money ("I'll take care of your car payment," he told her). Clearly he saw her role as including sex.

This chapter revealed how men view women in the workforce. Our conclusion is that men and their views vary just as much as do the women in the office. In the next chapter, we look at what women are thinking at the office.

8

What She Is Thinking

Give a man a free hand and he'll run it all over you.

Mae West

Feminism has remade the world of relationships, but not wholly to women's liking. Birth control allowed the woman to have more sexual partners, to become an equal in bed when it comes to enjoying sexual pleasure, and to be a single parent without stigma. Divorce lost its sting to a large extent, too, with sequential intimate relationships giving women a chance to try again for a more compatible partner. However, sexual "equality," where emotion is concerned, is often just a word. In the world of sexual equality, women are expected to have sex with a man without batting an eye. No strings attached? In the female psyche there are always "strings attached" because a woman is socialized to experience sex within the context of an emotionally secure relationship. Just "doing it" (which comes easy for the man) without some sort of involvement with the man is not what women are about. If sex often leaves the unmarried woman feeling bleak, hurt, or even used—as well as guilty for being needy or emotional—the office is an ideal place for her to see if she is in synch with a man.

The office provides a ballroom for getting acquainted with potential partners, à la Jane Austen, in a way that is amusing. Women invented etiquette in the first place, and they are always coming up with new hoops to put men through to see which candidate is the right one. However, the stakes are high. If a woman shows interest, and sees the person outside of work, she is vulnerable to sleep with that person, releasing the genie of passion from the bottle. And being in the lower rank at work, or having been so when she started out on her career, she is wary. A woman thinks, "I am more vulnerable than he is. It may be unwise to act on my impulse to go out with/sleep with him."

Taking the perspective of evolutionary biology, there is also an asymmetry between the sexes' desire to merge, where the man benefits from being a player and the woman is better off not letting herself get involved. As John Sparks writes of females in the mating game in *Battle of the Sexes: The Natural History of Sex*: "They are not, as usually portrayed, passive recipients of male lust, but are naturally cautious and highly discriminating . . . From their point of view, all males are different and, as every female wants only the very best possible specimen to father her offspring, she plays for time while assessing the quality of what is on offer."[1] While the male drops his sperm and moves on, females are fussy. Sparks gives the example of the courtship of the female guillemot (a kind of diving seabird): "She is on the lookout for the best father for her single chick—a healthy, assertive male, which can demonstrate his prowess at catching fish through courtship feeding." Similarly, the office female is the pretty young thing that looks for her best chances and does not settle for the first comer.

So women have their brakes on, and they have been inculcated with an air of nonchalance. At the same time, however, women know how to seduce. A woman keeps the strings of her violin tuned by flirting and preening, and is responsive when a man pleases her, especially if he is a realistic candidate for a sustained relationship. A woman knows that it's not a good idea to be too available to the man of her choice. It's natural (and advantageous) to a woman to maintain an air of mystique and keep him guessing. By this means she tests and increases his interest.

Women who have had sexual experience may know that they have orgasmic superiority. This means that they are comfortable with their bodies but also that they may be aware that virility in a partner is not something to be taken for granted. They wonder about each man—not the size of his shaft, which is a topic for jokes, but whether he is available as a lover because he can't perform in love and in life. Women will not mind getting some verbal affirmation that the man is heterosexual and has a healthy enjoyment of a consort in his bed. (Rather than tell tales, the man can demonstrate athletic energy and show some wistfulness about the conjugality he is missing at the moment).

Women are not beyond pampering a man's ego. This doesn't seem fake to a woman. Yet she will not present at the workplace as a doormat if she has a keen interest in a man since she knows she thrives better if she has his respect.

So, in general, women will conceal their interest in mating and give to the office guys the message, "I'm fine." They will also act more vulnerable than they are. They have a sense that men seem to like women who need to be rescued. Nevertheless, they know this is a dance, where they ask to be treated to the perks of a powerful male, but need their own ego strength, and need to keep him in line to assert a certain amount of independence. The male who displays his manly nature and charm, but proceeds with prudence, has the best chance with her.

HOW WOMEN SEE MEN

Some of the beliefs women have about men including the following:

1. Men are inconstant—they are skirt-chasers by nature. We know that men like to pursue. It stimulates a man's testosterone to go around half the world for us, whereas the man who is next door may hem and haw about whether he wants to proceed. Secondly, once the man has had us, he is spent and may cast us aside when his eye alights on another (never mind younger) woman, i.e., *If I can get her I wonder whom I can get.*
2. Men don't understand that a little romance is what women want. Heck, they don't even send Valentines past first grade! Men refer to other guys who do "dumb" romantic things, not realizing that we would adore a swain who carved our names into a tree trunk, wrote us a flowery inscription on a book of poetry, or gave us diamond earrings (regardless of the carets).
3. Men will do anything to have sex . . . in the beginning. When they are in courtship mode, they will buy us jewelry, treat us to expensive restaurants and vacations, and listen with fascination to what we say. Then, once we are in their beds, they would rather stay home and watch sports or play a video game. They interrupt our best stories with "So?" or even "What's the point?"
4. They are immature and out for a good time. Men we are dating like to pretend that we don't care about the future, or if they find us out thinking about the future, they will say, "Can't we just have a good time without asking where this is going?" They should realize that for us where sex is going, in the natural order of things, is having their babies and/or walking hand in hand into the sunset.
5. Sex is only an animal urge for men. That's why they fall asleep or hop up after they climax. They may be able to learn foreplay, but "afterplay"? Never! The male urge for sex is so different from the woman's that this statement expressed not just our perception but our validated experience time and time again. Men regard sex on the order of a good

workout or a delicious meal. Men have emotions but not about sex . . . it doesn't mean anything about a relationship or tomorrow.

6. Men get too wrapped up in technology. Men love their cars and computers and high-tech gadgets and they can look so silly with them. Listen to Jay Leno talk about working on his cars and you understand the essence of men and toys.

7. If given the chance, men are controlling. It is understandable, as they have more testosterone, and nature programmed them for more competition (for goods, territory and us). However, they also seem to try to dominate women as if they were suspicious of "the female principle"— as if they felt that women are question marks or wild cards. Women need space as men do. They can be "led" in a courteous slow dance, but find it hard to forgive men who ride roughshod over them, even once or twice. Men should realize that women have their competitive side as well.

8. Men calling women crazy is a cheap trick! How many axe murderers are women? And isn't it the secretive ones who are the worst criminals? Women are more emotional and prone to dramatics and tears. Men might grow up, get used to it, and get over it! If men could only learn that women are on the lookout for a man who appreciates their sincerity, and in flight from the ones who accuse them with words such as, "I don't want any outbursts," "You're PMS-ing" or "Don't act crazy."

9. A man will have little compunction about having two women at once. Many men seem to think of "job sharing" as when two women share him! If a woman calls a man on this he will soon comprehend that he has to choose one. However, he will start out by saying that he loves both women, and that they are just being possessive to expect him to have only one. Let him keep threesomes and nine-somes for his fantasies.

10. Married men are test-driven and more likely to be trained compared with bachelors. The stuffiest or most arrogant man is the one who has never married. Also, the man whose collar is yellow and whose cigarette ashes fall to the floor is the one who is still single. This, from the woman's view, is what "starter marriage" means, i.e., another woman worked his kinks out before he got to us.

11. Profit over people is a male way of thinking. Men have little interest in the social dimension of work in the way that women do. That's no problem, as women have more fun gossiping about men than if men joined in.

12. Men need women to teach them about where the relationship is heading. Men are going to dally forever. Women need to lead them along and teach them that sex isn't free, but rather means a relationship and commitment . . . Why is that so hard to understand?

HOW WOMEN SEE OTHER WOMEN AT THE OFFICE

- Status-seeker—She likes fellow employees to see that she is sought after.
- The woman who loves intrigue—She has a man in her life already but likes the flattery and the subterfuge/prospect of another love platter to spin at the office.
- Marriage-minded—Her biological clock means that she is not inclined to have a silly fling but that she is perked for love and insemination.
- Adventuress—Zipless sex is her stock in trade. She is in an experimental stage—which is short for most women.
- Cougar—She wants to prove that her beauty, allure, and youth are intact. She looks at every man who works under her as if he's a male centerfold.

WHAT WOMEN WANT FROM MEN IN AN OFFICE ROMANCE

The woman in the office romance needs reassurance that the man really likes her and that she isn't just a sexual target/dalliance. She needs to know that he is not talking with buddies about the relationship—that he is quite discreet about the fact that he is seeing her. She can't help acting differently from when they were just friends; she needs the man to understand her emotions, that she is higher keyed. She wonders if the man is able to move ahead both in the job and with her. She admires the man who can compartmentalize, by being friendly at work, and then letting her know how special she is when they are seeing each other that night.

She wants a sensitive partner who is comfortable to be with and treats her as an equal; however, if she meets him at work, she is going to see him against the backdrop of the other males. After French President Nicolas Sarkozy's advisors met Obama, he asked them *"Est-il faible?"* (Is he weak?). A head of state is naturally competitive with other heads of state, and Sarkozy wanted a report on the U.S. president's mettle. Being part of the work "jungle," the woman who meets the man in the workplace is hyperaware of whether he exerts power.

If a man lets a woman speak her mind, and doesn't try to make all the choices; if he communicates in an affable way about his feelings, and is patient when she just needs to vent (and doesn't always extend a solution); if he brings some heady romance and woos her, and can plan a future with her without getting defensive or shutting down, there is no competition. But to get to the point of being a lovely item, he has to make the correct dance steps. It's best to take into account both the "perfect impassivity" that a woman still feels she has to project toward the interested male at work, and the fact that she may tend to look at him critically, compared to the situation if they had met elsewhere, as though his résumé is a billboard he wears. As Olivia Judson, an evolutionary biologist, said, "Males evolve to control, females evolve to resist."[2]

Men to Avoid at the Office

I'm hungry, but not that hungry!
Melanie Griffith's character in the movie *Working Girl*

"My inner guidance system seems to take a hike the times I need it most (too scared to listen)," remarked one of the women we interviewed. I (Jane) have also had a lot of boyfriends, and have a suggestion or two about "who to avoid" on the romance road. I've been forced to make a getaway, and roadkill, both more than once. I also interviewed 50 single women about men they "should" have avoided. Leslie, a gorgeous interior decorator, was one of them. "Men to avoid? Hmm," she sighed. "I generally don't think in terms of who to avoid. Then again, this is why I'm single."

MEN TO AVOID

You know them and you've seen them. Here is a review:

The Office Flirt. He sees himself as a gift to the female gender. Stay away. Some people consume the opposite sex. They collect stripes. You'll be next, and discarded like the rest.

The One-Upper. This man wants to defeat you; perhaps because he doesn't like women, because he has a domineering mother, because the last woman rejected him—who knows? He will top your stories. If you took the wrong subway and ended up at Coney Island, he took the wrong plane and ended up in Portugal. His bettering you means that you are always in the one-down position. There's no equality here—stay away.

Mr. Ego. He's selling himself. He's not listening to you and he doesn't care. Mr. Ego will tell you about the places he's been, and the people he knows. He wants you to be impressed. It's all about him. Stay away.

Mr. Rebound. He's looking to park his heart (temporarily). He's either lost the love of his life, or his girlfriend is far away; he is in the mood for solace, or a transitional person. He is not settled and you won't be the one to settle him down.

The Uppity Guy. He lets you know he has a great future. He thinks people are stupid—it's his favorite word for them. He has pet names that bring everybody else in the organization down to the size that he's comfortable with. He is sarcastic.

The Worker with a Temper. Sometimes it seems "honest" for someone to fume and blow up at work. Once in a very great while is acceptable, but if he is blowing up on the job, where behavior is supposed to be in shades of beige, he may be emotionally violent in the private domain.

The Recently Separated. He's a wounded bird and brings out the nurturing in some women. But he's trouble. He's still in grief/ morning over what is not to be. It's better to let him heal on his own a bit than rescue him. He still feels like a married man and looks at the woman who sleeps with him as his mistress. Wait until the divorce is final—if it ever is.

The Barterer. He's the boss man or supervisor who treats you as his underling, and he's out to trade favors for sex. He feels important when he gives the flavor-of-the-month woman deferential treatment. You'll be shortchanged in the end and have to quit.

The Mystery Man. He doesn't tell you his address, his living circumstances, or his life goals, although he extracts yours. Even if he's as normal as can be, this is a sign of a very noncommittal type of man. Some are lured to this mystery. As George Orwell put it, "The moon is beautiful partly because we cannot reach it, the sea is impressive because one can never be sure of crossing it safely."[1]

The Career-Centrist. Some focus on career first, then marriage. They want to run for senator, reach partner in the firm, or win an Emmy for their show before they settle down 10 years from now. If you are on the same plan, no problem. Most women don't want to be one of his rides on the way to where he's going.

The Hyper Guy. This man cannot give you emotional security, not even for a third date, because he lives in a state of complex overdrive. He's wound up, distracted, and you will be another "issue" he has to deal with. Leave him to his own devices.

The Insanely Jealous Guy. No one person can satisfy our desire for friendship. The man who is miffed because you text your friends or are unavailable for lunch "today" is not for you. Next up, he will insist that you spend Thanksgiving with him, not your parents.

The Player. He flirts indiscriminately and has serial affairs, but sighs that you're the one he's been searching to find. In reality, he's out for a good time. Even if he does think you're "the one," someone else will catch his eye before you know it. You have nothing to offer him to settle him down—variety is his diet.

The Damaged One. This one has been through the meat grinder. The last woman had him for lunch, he was abandoned as a child, or his mother never loved him. Part of you can feel his pain. You think you can fill the void and help him find true happiness. He's very appealing—sensitive, with eyes that look into your soul; however, you are not going to be able to rescue him or fill that void. He needs to be in therapy—not in a relationship. Unless he wants to get help—and gets professional help—you won't have real intimacy with this man. A big part of him will always be "wed" to the pain.

The Older, Powerful Executive. Like it or not, he's a father figure and you're probably looking for the approval you never got. This is not a good prospect for a lasting relationship. You may get what you want at first, but most often differences loom too large. He likes you as a trophy, but has a hard time taking a lot of your concerns and interests seriously.

The Climber. This co-worker, like you, wants to get ahead, do well, have an interesting and good life—but he's more interested in how you can help him (disguised as "help each other") than in a romantic relationship. Romance is only the intro to "so what do you think?"

The Alcoholic. This guy lives a double life. He boozes when he is not at the office. For him, alcohol is not a choice but a necessity. He sneaks drinks (before he picks you up he downs two shots) and after he takes you home he will drink himself to sleep.

You won't be able to reach him. He's like Elvis—"I need the drugs, man."

Of course, any one of the above characteristics is not a deal breaker. Dear Abby is known for her advice, "Everyone comes with a catch." So no matter whom you select, there will be a personality characteristic, quirk, or something that turns you off, or that becomes a relationship challenge. And, of course, you have your own foibles that men must overlook and contend with.

CONTEXT CHANGES WHO THE PERSON IS

The behavior an individual engages in is always in reference to the context. The office context is the only backdrop against which you may have seen your man. Think of your schooldays or your children's. Kids behave differently at school and at home. The different contexts elicit different aspects of their personalities. The same goes for adults, so when you fall in love with a man you only know at the office, you are seeing one slice of the whole person, and it may not be a particularly representative slice. The fact that the context will determine the person you see necessitates dating the person long enough to get him out of the office to see who he is in different contexts—with your friends, with your family, interacting with his ex wife, grocery shopping, fixing a flat tire, and so on.

Perhaps the number one mistake women make is seeing only a part of someone—which is exactly what happens when we meet the opposite sex on the job. To know whether someone is going to be that special one, we have to go through all kinds of nice and delightful, and stressful and hard, experiences which show the other person unsheathed, and see whether we can do the dance of life together without smashing each other's toes. And you can't find out if your partner can dance if there is only one tune—the office. So, while we will identify men to avoid, it is important to change the job context to give you more information about this guy.

THE ROVING EYE TOPS ALL AS THE OFFICE MALE TO AVOID

The reason the man with the roving eye can be hard to spot at the office is that the motivation for his prowling mood isn't a loveless marriage or the lure of an adventure with a new woman, but his biological drive to have sex with different women, and the belief that he can do as he pleases. Tiger Woods, John Edwards, New York Governor Spitzer, South Carolina Governor Mark Sanford, and President Bill Clinton are guys who got caught with other women. They were also high-status, powerful males who felt that relationship rules do not apply to them. But, in the main, the roving eye men feel that something is missing.

Dr. Agnes Wilkie, a New York psychiatrist, notes that many people, men and women alike, upon reaching middle age undergo a review of their lives as lived thus far.[2] *They measure their progress in life against the goals and ideals they once held out for themselves when they began their lives as independent adults. When they look backward it is often disappointing and painful to acknowledge their failed dreams and view of themselves. Sometimes, people seek a chance to do it over, to, in essence, recapture their youthful idealized view of who they are. At a time when one's ascent in the world may be peaking or even starting to decline, it can be very appealing to look for ways to feel more powerful and valued.*

For some, this means challenging themselves to try new things: running a marathon; taking up an artistic endeavor; becoming a gourmet cook or a race car driver (Paul Newman, for example); buying a Jaguar convertible; or starting an affair. When men have invested themselves primarily in building their career, they may find that the relationships they share with their family may not be as close or rewarding as they would now like. In addition, they may not get the attention and deference at home that they are used to commanding at the office. When younger, perhaps more impressionable women catch their eye, it can be very appealing to try to recapture some youthful excitement, and turn away from one's disappointments, by engaging in an affair.

The younger woman, particularly in the office setting, may be the object of attention of several men simultaneously. This situation creates competition among the males. Younger men have youth, virility, and common age group interests to recommend them. Older males may offer a sense of worldliness, maturity, financial stability, protection, and material comforts. In the case of married men, the excitement of a clandestine affair adds a certain sexual charge to each encounter, whether public or private.

This can enhance the young woman's attraction to the older married man while it revives the man's sense of his own masculine appeal, sexuality, and youthfulness. All of this can enable him to avoid facing his own aging, and the intimations of mortality that come with it.

Dr. Wilkie's nuanced observations point up that all women who become the love object of a "midlife man" should be highly skeptical of the idea that "he needs me." For sure it's nonsense if he's married, because he is exploiting the woman as his mistress. He is going to control her, not give to her. If the new woman doesn't get holidays or weekends, she gets nothing. One affair that hit the press was between 48-year-old sports announcer Steve Phillips and a 22-year-old production assistant at the ESBN cable network where they both worked. The "other woman" started calling the wife after the breakup—graphically describing her husband's birthmarks. She also smashed her car against the stone posts of the Phillips home when leaving a letter for the wife, and confessed to having posed as a clandestine classmate of the teenage Phillips son to garner information about her inamorata.

What is telling (and also chilling) is how differently the lovers saw the affair. Phillips told the police that "This woman has clearly displayed erratic behavior and delusional tendencies," whereas his spurned lover said "I'm a real person in his life and I care deeply about his happiness" and that she was "sick of hiding." She clearly believed that she fulfilled his needs for love and understanding. Passion doesn't make us wise, but surely her sentiment that "we both can't have him" is a comprehensible one, even if her play for Phillips was over the top.

In one of the early treatises on the male midlife, *Crisis Time!: Love, Marriage and the Male at Midlife*, Dr. William A. Nolen concludes aptly: "The man in crisis is being foolish when he tries to reach back and reclaim the pleasures of his youth. He will almost certainly be better off if he clings to the less exciting but equally satisfying jobs of middle age; and, in most instances, with the wife partner who has gone through the turbulent younger years with him."[3] A theme of Andrew Young's book, *The Politician*, is the contrast between Rielle Hunter, presidential candidate John Edward's mistress (whom he met in a work context) and his wife of 30 years.[4] Rielle was the young adoring media whiz who was going to spin Edwards into stardom while his wife was at home tending the children.

THE SEPARATED MAN AT THE OFFICE: IS HE WORTH WAITING FOR?

In the realm of dating and mating in the workplace, getting past the impasse of a man's being tied (or welded) to a previous mate/ex-wife/mother of his child may be the most confusing problem women face—and the most prevalent. He is all yours during the workday, but you may not get together for seven days in a row when either of you has work demands. The woman at the office who is in love with the separated guy may tire of treading water until his divorce is final or spending a few hellish years while he is engaged in a custody battle with his former wife. The stories women told in our interviews differed, but the plight for those who love these part-time partners is the same: they get the short end of the stick. They give comfort to these beleaguered, often "stalled" men without getting financial, domestic, or full emotional support in return. They pin hopes on a dream of the future and make do with a thin present. They are forced as a third party into the man's prior relationship, when they only want to build with love and positive energy their own new relationship.

Phyllis, a college administrator said: *The ties to his ex were lethal live wires. I was caught in the put-down position, screwed over for years. I actually prided myself on being long suffering. If his wife needed him so she could go out for an evening, he would cancel with me at the last minute—and expect me to admire him as a good daddy. He was more a spineless pawn. I felt powerless. Sometimes I lashed out. Then I began listening to what he said when I was angry, that if I wasn't content with him, I should find someone who could make me happy. One day the light bulb went on and I started to redress my inertia by extending my social range, including seeing other men."*

Here's another example: Leon, a physician, has had a series of affairs with receptionists. Separated from his wife, and unwilling to sell his summer home and the plane that takes him there, he says he loves intimacy and women but is always between girlfriends. *I look at him, in his 50s, and think he is old to think he can cheat Venus like this. Autonomy, prestige, and science brought him into medicine, and he is keeping his autonomy by a convenient marital status and unavailability to his serial girlfriends.*

And who are you? You are passionate . . . you are sticking it out. You're feeling carefree or you had a whiff of the complications from seeing him rant on his cell phone leaving the office. You are adaptable. You manage. Do you want to end up with the icing, not the cake, or do you have a piece of the cake when you want and deserve the whole thing? Or is it his should-be-irrelevant ex-wife, whose demands on him as the father of her children act like a thousand ropes on a hot air balloon that keep carrying him away? In whatever way he is mixed up with a former love partner, you are sharing this man as a consequence.

The woman who is emotionally involved with someone who turns out to have a private life that still has claims on him (or claws into him) needs to be strong and upbeat, value herself, and develop some strategies. She needs to keep her eyes on the shore and her oars in the oarlocks. There is a Finnish saying that the woman is the neck, and the man is the head, and the neck turns the head.

Stay mindful of your needs and your goal (to change the relationship from part-time to full-time, or to bail). It is important to understand what the man is going through. He may be temporarily insensitive and withholding, but still be, as we women secretly will remark, "good material." He is having trouble closing the door on his old relationship, so don't you put your foot in the door and mix it up with him on this. He may have trouble resolving personal dilemmas in general . . . but you can't solve them for him. He may have been betrayed by his former partner and be more invested in revenge than moving ahead with you. See if he settles down, don't analyze him to him. He may be a bit of a tortoise but love you, so don't despair if the process of becoming a true couple takes longer than you had expected.

Or, he may have huge intimacy issues, secretly get an ego boost from letting you hang on a limb, and neurotically maintain his prerogative to control everything in his life, including you. He may have a mother who told him that he can do no wrong . . . and he still believes it, viz., he can mistreat or mislead you without conscience.

Rebecca worked for the publicist of a performer who is a household name. She helped throw a party at his house. He told her she was better than a wife (he was divorced), and she and he swam naked in his pool after the other guests left. One thing led to another. *I was flattered that he pursed a quiet sparrow like me. He thought I was cosmopolitan and unconventional, so I wouldn't mind being secreted from limousine to plane wearing a scarf and dark glasses for our trip abroad. Here was a man who had ruined his marriage and created a philosophy around it, where the mistress was treated like a princess except she had to leave by the back stairs. Once he saw me talking to another man, and he panicked he would lose me. That was because he had little as a person to give. He faulted me for it and I wanted to end the affair. That's when he said, "You can't. You work for me. I'll see you lose your job." That was true in a way, as he was a major client, but I called his bluff and wouldn't see him alone again. He didn't carry out his threat.*

AVOIDANCE AS A PROTOCOL

If you don't want one of the men identified above (even though you have flirted with him), limit your interactions as much as possible. Remember: your reputation is your biggest asset, even though it doesn't appear on your résumé. We like the advice of a management consultant: "Dealing with bad guys does seem a bit dicey, doesn't it? The important common denominator . . . is that whatever we do, we do without malicious intent. If we cross that border into *bad guy* activities, we can drag ourselves down to the lowest common denominator and can become bad guys, like our untrustworthy foes."[5]

10

Men to Include in Your Office Search

The man you eliminate from consideration is the same one who could be the love of your life.

Anonymous

Marie Sklodowska aced her studies and was living in a six-story walkup in Paris. She had been hired by an institute to test the magnetic properties of various steels but the Sorbonne's physics laboratory was too crowded to contain her equipment. A professor friend of Marie's introduced her to someone he thought could help her. It seems to have been love at first sight. She noted his open expression and noble air of detachment. He and she both had had rocky prior relationships. She turned down his initial proposal of marriage, as she felt obliged to return to her native Poland after concluding her studies. Biographer Denis Brian[1] tells how Pierre found an apartment with two separate units where they could be platonic working partners, as Marie didn't love him enough to marry him. This was the beginning of an inseparable work and love relationship between Marie and Pierre Curie (they eventually married), winners of the Nobel Prize and discoverers of radium.

While Marie was more focused on her work than on finding a man, women of today are more likely to scan the workplace for potential partners, eliminating some and engaging others. Most women in the workplace complain that "there's no one out there—all the good ones are gone." Some look without seeing that the cultural printout of "tall, dark, and handsome" does not always appear (and even if he does, he may not make a good partner/spouse). In this chapter, we emphasize the importance of looking closely at the prospects at hand.

WHERE THE BOYS ARE

The workplace most conducive to finding a partner is where there are many co-workers at equal level, where the work involves and doesn't frown on conversing, and where there is an on-site cafeteria or where people gather to talk before or after work.

Some work roles are dominated by one gender over the other. Women are overrepresented as secretaries, nurses, elementary school teachers, and day care workers and men as electricians, bricklayers, carpenters, and in the armed forces. Few women will enter an "all-male profession" just to land a mate. Rather, they will look among the options where they are.

NUMBER OF SINGLE/DIVORCED WOMEN LOOKING FOR PARTNERS

There are 26 million adult women who have never married and 14 million divorced women in the United States.[2] Since over 96 percent of those who have never married will eventually marry[3] (as will over three-quarters of the divorced women), their goal is often the same: to find a man, a companion with whom to share their life/have kids (or share the parenting of existing children). They've lived their life in the prescribed order—education, economic independence, career, dating. They are exhausted from looking for a man and upset about being alone . . . So, where is "he"? Closer than you think.

TO FIND A PARTNER—LOOK OUTSIDE THE BOX

It is advantageous when seeking a mate to widen the scope from one's previous criteria of who is traditionally suitable and proper to include those of a different race, age, religion, country of origin, education, economic status, and physical appearance. One of the people we interviewed told us that "Women eliminate from consideration men who could be the love of their life. I know. I ended up with a guy unlike any I would ever have imagined (racial, age, religious differences) yet we connect on core values and have the emotional closeness everyone wants."

Indeed, the person who gets stuck on and weds the person whom others admire for his "appropriateness" ("Everybody liked him but me," said one of the women we interviewed) but who is left with the sense that something is awry and hollow is missing the boat of possibilities. If you take an open-minded and openhearted approach to dating people your circle of friends might not match you up with, you will instantly have an untapped pool of eligible and desirable single partners.

Somebody you overlook because of some conventional category in your head may/could be the man or woman of your dreams. We all have prejudices. Our life experience erodes these biases, but it takes a long time, possibly a lifetime, whereas we want to resolve the question of pairing off much sooner. How do you see a person's worth without being put off by the trappings of the unfamiliar? How do you negotiate the getting-to-know-you and dating process so there aren't misunderstandings? What can you expect to be the way stations on the course to true reciprocal lasting love?

Put on new glasses—hey, we elected Barack Obama as our President! Maybe your aunt or mother would not have exchanged glances with men of a different ethnicity, or with less education, or with a child in tow. But you are free to go out with someone who watches an Urdu or Finnish play-by-play of the world cup, or has a mother who wears a sari, or puts himself through college by being the translator on his crew of Brazilian masons. Interracial dating today is commonplace. In our multicultural, pluralistic society, people everywhere are different from the stereotype who is of the "right" age, race, religion, etc. We should not be put off by the fact that her family celebrates the holidays differently or that he has a child and discusses parenting with an ex. Instead, focus on whether the person likes you, shows an interest in a relationship with you, is kind, is supportive of your interests, has character, works hard, loves his family, is open to new ideas, and is charitable and optimistic. Only if you look beyond skin color, age, accent, ethnic roots, the house of worship someone attends, and the amount of formal education the person has attained can you know if these factors matter at all. The person you eliminate is the very person with whom you could have electric chemistry and share a wonderful durable life/marriage/family. And this person may love you as no other man has.

The reality of finding a mate is that there are a limited number of heterosexual, unmarried/unpartnered men of your color, age, religion, and educational background. If you keep your eyes open for the appealing person, e.g., the guy in the mailroom who is putting himself through an MBA program, you open up new possibilities and may be looking at your prince.

Meeting Scott did much more than change Molly's status from single to married. Both of them worked for a Route 128 high-tech company outside Boston. Both came from small towns, had one parent who taught high school math, were 36, loved to sail and played in amateur chamber groups. What was dissimilar and might have kept them apart was that Scott is African American and Molly is white. There is a force field around them as a couple. With new zest from their relationship, Scott took a woodworking course, made a roll-top desk for Molly's birthday, and found a career he loved—cabinetry. They are building a sailboat together. "We'll learn how to sail after it's done," said Scott with his typical ironic humor. Said Molly: *Scott and I are one of those couples who were born for each other, but we are shy, and maybe if we hadn't worked together, the skin thing would have been another excuse to stay at a polite distance.*

The advantage of developing a friendship in the workplace is that prejudice melts with exposure. Why let the good one get away just because his family tree was separated from yours a couple of hundred thousand years ago, or because he wasn't born in the same decade or country? Become more open so that you can respond to the worthy guy who genuinely likes you, but who isn't what you expected when you played with Barbie and Ken, the matching set. Singles of any age (but particularly women 30, 40, or older) can rethink their "He's got to be at least 5'11, be four years older/younger, and have the same race, religion, and ethnic and educational background as mine." Look outside the box. Instead of regular Wonder Bread, today's men are pita or lavish, foccacia or dark rye—new tastes that have become "our tastes" because of America's new diversity and pluralism. Some of the women we interviewed opened their minds and hearts to a mate outside her own ideal notions. We now look at three areas: race, age, and religion.

INTERRACIAL RELATIONSHIPS AND MARRIAGES

The workplace is the optimal context to rethink previous notions and find your man without reference to skin color. Depending on one's own race, being open to an office romance with someone from a different racial background provides an array of options: American white, American black, Caribbean black, African black, Indian, Chinese,

Japanese, Korean, Mexican, Malaysian, and Hindu mates. Only a few cross racial lines to marry: less than five percent of the 60 million marriages in the United States are interracial.[4]

While the standard explanations for low rates of interracial marriage are racial prejudice and discrimination, a third explanation is exposure—people of different racial backgrounds do not live next to each other, go to the same school, or worship in the same place. The workplace is one of the few places where the races have the opportunity to learn about each other.

Those who venture to cross racial lines are more likely to have been married before, to be age-discrepant, to live far away from their parents, to have been reared in racially tolerant homes, and to have continued their education past high school. Some may also belong to religions that encourage interracial unions. The Baha'i religion, which has more than 6 million members worldwide and 84,000 in the United States, teaches that God is particularly pleased with interracial unions. Finally, interracial spouses may tend to seek contexts of diversity. "I was reared in a military family, have been everywhere, and have met people of different races and nationalities throughout my life. I seek diversity," noted one of the persons we interviewed.

Getting involved with someone of another race in the office will have its challenges. Black people partnered with white people have their blackness and racial identity challenged by other black people. White people partnered with black people may lose their white status and have their awareness of whiteness heightened more than ever before. Moreover, the partner in an interracial relationship is not given full status as a member of the other partner's race.[5]

Black-white partnering also varies depending on color and gender. Two researchers[6] found that the pairing of a black male and a white female is regarded as "less appropriate" than that of a white male and a black female. In the former, the black male "often is perceived as attaining higher social status (i.e., the white woman is viewed as the black man's 'prize,' stolen from the more deserving white man)." In the latter, when a white male pairs with a black female, "no fundamental change in power within the American social structure is perceived as taking place." Don't expect it to be easy. In one study of adolescents who were dating cross racially, disapproval from peers was reported.[7] The workplace may have older, more mature adults . . . but don't count on an absence of racism.

Black-white interracial marriages are likely to increase—slowly. Not only has white prejudice against African Americans in general

SELF-TEST: Attitudes Toward Interracial Dating Scale

Interracial dating or marrying is when two people from different races date or marry. This test will allow you to find out your openness to dating and marrying across racial lines. Read each item carefully, and in each space, write a number from 1 to 7. The lower the number, the more you disagree; the higher the number, the more you agree. There are no right or wrong answers to any of these statements.

1	2	3	4	5	6	7
Strongly Disagree						Strongly Agree

____1. I believe that interracial couples date outside their race to get attention.

____2. I feel that interracial couples have little in common.

____3. When I see an interracial couple, I find myself evaluating them negatively.

____4. People date outside their own race because they feel inferior.

____5. Dating interracially shows a lack of respect for one's own race.

____6. I would be upset with a family member who dated outside our race.

____7. I would be upset with a close friend who dated outside our race.

____8. I feel uneasy around an interracial couple.

____9. People of different races should associate only in nondating settings.

____10. I am offended when I see an interracial couple.

____11. Interracial couples are more likely to have low self-esteem.

____12. Interracial dating interferes with my fundamental beliefs.

____13. People should date only within their race.

____14. I dislike seeing interracial couples together.

____15. I would not pursue a relationship with someone of a different race, regardless of my feelings for that person.

____16. Interracial dating interferes with my concept of cultural identity.

____17. I support dating between people with the same skin color, but not different skin color.

____18. I can imagine myself in a long-term relationship with someone of another race.

____19. As long as the people involved love each other, I do not have a problem with interracial dating.

____20. I think interracial dating is a good thing.

SCORING

First, reverse the numbers you wrote down for items 18, 19, and 20 by switching them to the opposite side of the spectrum. For example, if you selected 7 for item 18, replace it with a 1; if you selected 3, replace it with a 5, and so on. Next, add your scores and divide by 20. Possible final scores range from 1 to 7, with 1 representing the most positive attitudes toward interracial dating and 7 representing the most negative attitudes toward interracial dating.

HOW OTHERS SCORED

113 males and 200 females took the Attitudes Toward Interracial Dating Scale (IRDS). The average score on the IRDS was 2.88. Scores ranged from 1.00 to 6.60, suggesting very positive views of interracial dating. Men scored an average of 2.97; women an average of 2.84.

Source: The Attitudes Toward Interracial Dating Scale, 2004. Mark Whatley, Ph.D., Department of Psychology, Valdosta State University, Valdosta, GA 31698. The scale is used by Dr. Whatley's permission.

declined, but segregation in school, at work, and in housing has also decreased, permitting greater contact between the races. The above self-test allows you to find out the degree to which you are open to involvement in an interracial relationship.

AGE-DISCREPANT RELATIONSHIPS AND MARRIAGES

A less controversial and more frequent outside-the-box office romance is the age-discrepant relationship. In marriage, these are referred to as ADMs (age-dissimilar marriages), in contrast to ASMs (age-similar marriages). ADMs are also known as May-December marriages. Typically, the woman is in the spring of her youth (May) whereas the man is in the later years of his life (December). There have been a number of May-December celebrity marriages, including that of Celine Dion, who is 26 years younger than René Angelil (in 2011, aged 43 and 69). Larry King is also 26 years older than his seventh wife, Shawn (in 2011, he was 76). Michael Douglas is 25 years older than his wife, Catherine Zeta Jones. Ellen DeGeneres is 15 years older than Portia de Rossi, her partner (they "married" in 2008).

One might assume that these marriages are less happy because the spouses were born into such different age contexts. Research shows otherwise. Two researchers[8] compared 35 ADMs (in which spouses were 14 or more years apart) and 35 ASMs (in which spouses were less than 5 years apart) and found no difference in reported marital satisfaction between the two groups. As is true in other research, wives reported lower marital satisfaction and more household responsibilities in both groups.

Perhaps the best example of a May-December marriage that "worked" is that of Oona and Charles Chaplin. She married him at age 18 (he was 54). Their May-December alliance was expected to last the requisite six months, but they remained married for 35 years and raised eight children.

Although less common, in some age-discrepant relationships the woman is older than her partner. Mary Tyler Moore is 18 years older than her husband, Robert Levine; they have been married 25 years. Demi Moore is 16 years older than her husband, Ashton Kutcher (she was 40 and he was 27 when they wed). Valerie Gibson is the author of *Cougar: A Guide for Older Women Dating Younger Men*. She noted that the current use of the term "cougars" refers to "women, usually in their 30s and 40s, who are financially stable and mentally independent and looking for a younger man to have fun with." Gibson noted that one-third of women between the ages of 40 and 60 date younger men. Financially independent women need not select a man in reference to his breadwinning capabilities. Instead, these "cougars" are looking for men perhaps to marry, but definitely to enjoy. The downside of such relationships comes if when the commitment becomes serious he wants to have children, which may spell the end of the relationship.

INTERRELIGIOUS RELATIONSHIPS AND MARRIAGE

More frequent than out-of-the-box racial and age-discrepant relationships are interreligious relationships. Indeed, almost 40 percent (37%) of the marriages in the United States are interreligious.[9]

Are people in interreligious marriages less satisfied with their marriages than those who marry someone of the same faith? The answer depends on a number of factors. First, people in marriages in which one or both spouses profess "no religion" tend to report lower levels of marital satisfaction than those in which at least one spouse has a religious tie. People with no religion are often more liberal and less bound by traditional societal norms and values; they feel less constrained to stay married for reasons of social propriety.

The impact of a mixed religious marriage may also depend more on the devoutness of the partners than on the fact that the partners are of different religions. If both spouses are devout in their religious beliefs, they may expect some problems in the relationship (although not necessarily). Less problematic is the relationship in which one spouse is devout but the partner is not. If neither spouse in an interfaith marriage is devout, problems regarding religious differences may be minimal or nonexistent. In their marriage vows, one interfaith married couple (he is Christian, she is Jewish) said that they viewed their different religions as an opportunity to strengthen their connections to their respective faiths and to each other. "Our marriage ceremony seeks to celebrate both the Jewish and Christian traditions, just as we plan to in our life together," the couple said in their wedding vows.

CROSS-NATIONAL RELATIONSHIPS AND MARRIAGES

The workplace is ripe with opportunities for employees to meet someone born in another country. Over 38 million foreign-born people live in the United States: most are from Latin America (20 million); others hail from Europe and Asia.[10] There is an openness (particularly among college students) among people in the United States to marry someone from another country: In a study of 1,319 college students, 60.4 percent reported that they would be willing to do so.[11]

Some people from foreign countries marry an American citizen to gain U.S. citizenship, but immigration laws now require the marriage to last two years before citizenship is granted. If the marriage ends before two years, the foreigner must prove good faith (that the marriage was not just to gain entry into the country) or he or she will be asked to leave the country.

As with any potential mate, it is important to learn about the cultural values of a person who was brought up in another country. More often than not, his cultural mores will prevail and clash strongly with his American bride's expectations, especially if the couple should return to his country. One American female described her experience of marriage to a Pakistani, who violated his parents' wishes by not marrying the bride they had chosen for him in childhood. The couple had two children before the four of them returned to Pakistan. The woman felt that her in-laws did not accept her and were hostile toward her. They also imposed their religious beliefs on her children and took control of their upbringing. When this situation became intolerable, the woman wanted to return to the United States. Because the children were viewed as being "owned" by their father, she was not allowed to take them with her and was banned from even seeing them. This woman had met her husband while in college. Like many international students, he was from a wealthy, high-status family; the woman was powerless to fight the family. The woman has not seen her children in six years.

Cultural differences do not necessarily cause stress in cross-national marriage. If such stress exists, it often results from society's intolerance of the marriage, as manifested in attitudes of friends and family. Japan and Korea place an extraordinarily high value on racial purity. At the other extreme is the racial tolerance evident in Hawaii, where a great number of out-group marriage is normative.

There are other aspects of office romances worthy of our consideration in addition to these interracial, age-discrepant, interreligious, and cross-national romances examples. They include:

Education: Should it really matter how educated he is or where he went to school? Isn't it more pertinent that he has common sense and treats you with respect? Sometimes it's a sign of strength to hold a decent job, which you have learned hands-on. Not everyone has the patience or economics for the college years.

Previous marital status/children: It is common for men in their mid-30s to have been married/had a child. Eliminate them from consideration, and there goes half of your pool of eligible men.

Personal Appearance: How "cute" does he need to be? Unfortunately, this is often a deal breaker, but it prevents us from finding true love. It's too bad, especially since there are so many "odd" couples who have stayed together happily long after the so-called "perfectly matched beauties" have split up.

Economic Status: Who cares if he earns a few dollars less than you? In this economy, it's a miracle if he has a job. More important is that he has skills and develops them.

And, there are nerds.

NERDS: THE OFTEN OVERLOOKED POSSIBILITY

In the classic Brothers Grimm fairy tale, *The Princess and the Frog*, Prince Charming is hiding in the form of a frog. The princess must step outside of her typical dating schema and place her trust in the frog. After a kiss, she is rewarded with happily ever after—a prince with whom she falls in love and who loves her. Even before she realizes that he's her one and only, the frog is the kind of helpmeet every princess needs. When the princess drops her golden ball in the well, the frog is affected by her tears and makes things better. While applying the wisdom of a fairy tale requires caution, when a woman is in a stage of potentiality for a relationship—perhaps single and playing some sort of metaphorical catch in the garden/woods of her workplace—she can keep her eyes open for a man who is neither surface-handsome nor the life of the party. He may not have the sheen to dazzle her friends, but instead has real character, self-restraint, and a kindness that can bring a good woman her complement and happiness. In essence, a nerd is often a shining prince masquerading as a frog, which a woman might consider as a potential partner, and who is (psychologically) waiting there for romance to transform him (with her) into lifelong lovers.

A "nerd" is usually regarded as someone who is socially inept but very accomplished at some scientific or technical endeavor. Nerds, sometimes known as "geeks," are typically well-versed in computers and play video games. This is the guy in the office who is always on time, has an awkward smile, and wears the same sweater three days in a row. Nerds are often discounted as potential partners either because of their lack of social skills or because they choose not to compete with other males in the social arena. "Look again," says Leia, who married a nerd and says they are the untapped market of great husbands.

Nerds are romantic and appreciative of attention. My husband absolutely adores me. He looks to see how he can please me, like rubbing my feet, cooking, or doing the dishes. And talk about support. I needed to make a career move and he did not hesitate to facilitate the change. Of course, our relationship is not a one-way street. I am deliriously in love with my man. He's handsome, bright, fun, and understands my quirkiness, too.

If you're looking for nerds around the office, here are a few tips on locating your hidden prince charming: They could be in accounting, information technology services, or even within your own field. They may be very efficient and great at their job, even to the point of not being talkative with their co-workers. Don't mistake this for lack of interest; instead look at this quality as a devotion to their work. If you are looking for someone who can show a considerable amount of commitment, these nerds should be the frogs you're looking to kiss.[12]

Nerds are for when a woman is ready to pair up, and that may be a change in her outlook, where the fun guy or crazy artist was just right for the ski weekend or when you moved to the city and are getting your bearings.

TAKING THE ROAD NOT TRAVELED

Whom have you inadvertently eliminated as a potential partner on the basis of their race, age, religion, country of origin, or nerdiness? Reevaluate these men! The first date will likely differ from dating someone who is not that different from you. Your differences will create important questions and provide tips for early meetings. Can you talk about the differences? You are going to need to do a lot of watching and listening.

How will your dating and marrying someone outside the box "go down" with friends and family? Your friends can sometimes be more objective than you can, and will tell you if you are suited to one another on more than superficial grounds. It is also significant that friends are generally accepting and positive about such relationships. They can be your support system. It's your family who can drag you down.

Don't take warnings to beware of men who are fond of "Asian women" or "cute blonds," or "Mexican women" because they have fantasies about subservient demure wives at face value—instead, learn for yourself about his traditions and his life view. He is not his family any more than you are yours.

The theme of this chapter is to be open about whom you consider a potential partner. We are all socialized to reject certain categories of people out of hand. But look again. Behind the demographics of a person may very well be a loving, respectful, lifetime partner. If you don't look, you won't see.

11

Should You Marry Your Office Love?

Keep your eyes wide open before marriage, half shut afterwards.

Ben Franklin

So, you're in love. You've found someone with whom you have chemistry and are aboard the love train moving toward commitment and marriage. Almost a third (32%) of the 5,231 employees in the Career Builders.com survey reported that they went on to marry the person they had dated at work.[1] Before making the transition from office lovers to spouses, carefully evaluate your partner and your relationship. In this chapter, we review how you can transfer your love at the office into a happy and enduring relationship when you get him home.

PERSONAL QUALITIES THAT PREDICT A HAPPY, DURABLE FUTURE

The following is a list of qualities associated with the kind of partner who ends up in a happy, enduring relationship. People with these qualities bring "something to the relationship table" that is valuable for their years ahead in a relationship. We have not listed these in the order of importance.

1. Supportive rather than controlling. The behavior that today's women *hate* in a man is that he is controlling—about what she does, where she goes, what she wears. Such a quality is predictive of a disastrous future. The opposite behavior is supportive—of your interests, values, and goals. Whatever you are interested in or excited by, he likes it, encourages it, and will drive you there if you need a ride. How do you

know if a guy is supportive or not? The best answer is to run the clock on your relationship. About two years of friendship segueing to courtship is best so that you have an opportunity to observe the degree to which he supports your interests. Such support is a quality that will endear him to you and predicts a wonderful future.

2. Optimistic rather than pessimistic. Spouses who look on the bright side of everything are associated with happy and durable marriages, just as pessimists are to be avoided.[2] The latter will find something wrong with everything—the job, the new car, and you. A person's view also affects his or her mood. Optimists are happy, enthusiastic, and resilient. Pessimists find little joy in anything and expect rain in the afternoon. The Roman poet Ovid said, "Before you run in double harness, look well to the other horse." Make sure you link with someone who sees the sunrise and the potential for great things, and believes that everything will work out. Such a perspective is important, since it is not the events in life that make us happy or sad, but our view of them.

3. "Other-focused" rather than narcissistic.[3] One of the central elements of love is that it engenders a genuine concern for the well-being of one's partner, sometimes to the exclusion of one's own needs. A couple was grieving over the death of their small dog of 15 years. The husband was interested in a new, black 60-pound Labrador retriever that was being made available to the couple if they wanted it. In fact, he said the new dog would be "perfect." The wife did not like the size or color of the Lab, but since the husband was so taken by the animal, she acquiesced to their getting the dog—she ended up being as bonded to the dog as her husband. She derived pleasure in her partner's joy: this is the quality that spouses should look for in each other. Narcissistic individuals are like four-year olds—they see everything from their point of view and the needs of others are irrelevant.

4. High frequency of positives rather than negatives.[4] A deliriously happy spouse is usually one who loves his or her partner, feels "cherished" by the partner and is the recipient of a high frequency of positive verbal and nonverbal behaviors. Positive verbal behavior includes, "I love you," "You are terrific," "You are beautiful," etc. Positive nonverbal behavior may include backrubs, going out to dinner, and taking over some task that poses some difficulty for the other person.

   It is important that the high frequency of positives occur in the context of no negatives, as one barb ("Those pants make you look fat") can offset 20 positives. Indeed, a high frequency of negatives qualifies as abuse and should eliminate a partner from serious consideration. Such negatives will only increase in marriage, so end the relationship, now.

5. Responsible rather than impulsive.[5] A mature/steady partner is one you can count on to be responsible rather than impulsive. Jill needed to be away from home for a weekend to take care of her aging father.

Her husband promised to paint the garage while she was gone. Then her husband's old Army buddy from Iraq came by while Jill was gone, and they ended up drinking all weekend and trashing the house. Her husband's impulsiveness also evidenced in his not being able to stay focused on his job or schoolwork (he was taking online courses). Jill felt that she could not count on him for anything. A lack of impulse control is problematic in relationships, since the impulsive person is less likely to consider the consequences of his or her actions. For example, to some people, having an affair might seem harmless; however, it typically has devastating consequences for the partners and the relationship.

6. Secure rather than hypersensitive. Hypersensitivity to perceived criticism means that one gets hurt easily. Any negative statement or criticism is received with a greater impact than the partner intended. The disadvantage of such hypersensitivity is that a partner may learn not to give feedback for fear of hurting the hypersensitive partner. Such a lack of feedback to the hypersensitive partner blocks information about what the person does that upsets the other and what could be done to make things better. Hence, the hypersensitive person has no way of learning that something is wrong, and the partner has no way of alerting the hypersensitive partner. The result is a relationship in which the partners can't talk about what is wrong, so the potential for change is limited.

7. Positive self-concept but not inflated ego.[6] It is important to select a partner who feels good about himself but who does not have an inflated ego. Such an ego is an exaggerated sense of oneself that may translate into denigrating the other ("Since I'm so great, you're not"). A person with an inflated sense of self may also be less likely to consider the other person's opinion in negotiating a conflict and prefer to dictate an outcome. Such disrespect for the partner will be devastating to the relationship.

8. Flexible rather than perfectionist.[7] Perfectionists may require perfection of themselves *and* others. Everyone must be on time, the house must be spotless, and the children must earn all As from kindergarten on. Such a view is destined to create relationship problems, since the world is not perfect and neither are the people in it.

9. Secure emotional attachments rather than insecure attachments.[8] Having been loved/cared for by one's parents creates a strong sense of emotional comfort/security. In general, someone who was not loved as a child tends to be insecure, suspicious, jealous . . . indeed, a wreck. Pick a partner with strong family connections. This will help to ensure strong emotional bonding with you, which predicts a very intimate relationship.

10. Independent of parents rather than controlled by parents. Individuals who are controlled by someone, perhaps their parents, grandparents, former partner, or child, compromise the marriage relationship because their allegiance is external to the couple's relationship. Unless the person is able to break free of such control, the ability to make independent

decisions will be thwarted, which will both frustrate the spouse and challenge the partner/marriage.

11. Faithful and honest. Yeah, right! Where are you going to find a guy who is both? Everywhere is the answer. Just as there are womanizers who have been with hundreds of women (and more to come), there are true blue men who have been very selective and completely faithful in each of their relationships before they met you. And they will be faithful to you, too. How will you know if you have a true blue guy? His track record is the greatest predictor. If he has a history of infidelity, lots of women, and lying, it is doubtful if he will be any different with you.

The character of Don Draper, from the television drama *Mad Men*, exemplifies of a man who has a track record of affairs and deceit. In three seasons, he had three affairs. Meanwhile, he had been married before (which his wife did not know about) and was actually someone else (he just assumed the name and "life" of a guy named Don Draper)—not a good bet for fidelity in a relationship. Meanwhile his wife Betty had her own dalliances—flirting with guys, kissing them, and having sex (and getting pregnant) with a stranger. Do these two deserve each other?

PERSONALITY TYPES TO AVOID IN TURNING AN OFFICE LOVER INTO A SPOUSE

In addition to various personal qualities to avoid in selecting your man, Table 11.1 reflects some particularly troublesome personality types you could meet at the office or workplace that do not bode well for being a good marital partner.

RELATIONSHIP QUALITIES THAT PREDICT A GREAT MARRIAGE

Having asked yourself if your potential partner has the personal qualities that make for a good spouse, and having identified personality types to avoid, we now look at relationship qualities that predict a good marriage. As a couple, do you and your office partner have the type of relationship that will make for a happy and durable Mr. and Mrs.? One of the best ways to know if your relationship has such qualities is to look at the spouses in marriages that last to discover some of the facts and myths of such relationships.

Table 11.1   Personality Types That Make Bad Spouses

Type	Characteristics	Impact on You
Paranoid	Suspicious, distrustful, thin-skinned, defensive	You may be accused of everything.
Schizoid	Cold, aloof, solitary, reclusive	You may feel that you can never "connect," and that the person does not return your love.
Borderline	Moody, unstable, volatile, unreliable, suicidal, impulsive	You never know what your Jekyll-and-Hyde partner will be like, which could be dangerous.
Antisocial	Deceptive, untrustworthy, conscienceless, remorseless	This person will cheat on you, lie, and not feel guilty.
Dependent	Helpless, weak, clingy, insecure	This person will demand your full time and attention; your other interests will incite jealousy.
Obsessive-compulsive	Rigid, inflexible	This person has rigid ideas about how you should think and behave and may try to impose them on you.

They Are Committed to Making Their Marriage Work

Couples who stay married are determined to do so. They value themselves, their vows, and their relationship, and they intend to overcome whatever problems they encounter. There is no back door. "Marriage isn't fun at times," says one spouse who has been married for 26 years, "but you've got to look at it as something you and your partner work on together and are committed to. If you don't feel that way you won't make it."

They Spend Time Together

"I slept and dreamed that life was beauty. I woke and found that life was duty," wrote Ellen Hooper, a nineteenth-century poet. Were marriage the same romantic whirl of courtship, all couples would stay together. But the demands of careers and children inevitably cut into the time that spouses have for each other. Those who stay together continue to make time for each other. Just as there are laws of science (such as gravity), there are laws of relationships. And one of the great laws of marriage is that if the partners don't have time for each other, they won't have a relationship.

They Communicate Effectively

The cliché that "good communication is the most important part of a successful marriage" is true. Good communication means talking with your partner about what you think and feel, being interested in what your partner says, and discussing conflicts/resolving issues in a way that neither partner feels belittled or attacked. But the real value of communication is that it provides an emotional connection between the partners.

They Are Skillful at Negotiating Compromises

Being skillful at negotiating compromises is part of good communication. Regardless of how much spouses are in love with each other, they will disagree. Such disagreement is healthy because it represents a mutual willingness to express preferences. Spouses who do not tell their partners that they are unhappy may grow bitter and communicate their hostility in more subtle ways, such as alcohol abuse and withdrawal of affection. By making their preferences known to each other, spouses can negotiate and compromise their differences. Not to resolve conflicts is to keep the conflicts alive in the relationship. If we do not solve our problems, they get worse.

But we are a bit clumsy at negotiating compromises. We tend to get defensive, want our own way, and try to control our partner. Negotiating and compromising require an entirely different set of responses—and couples in marriages that last have learned them. Two examples of conflict and how they were resolved follow:

- She wanted him to go to church with her and he wanted to sleep in. Result: He went to church with her that morning and she helped him fill the vending machines (his job) with new products that afternoon (he normally had to fill the machines alone on Sunday afternoon).
- He wanted her to go with him to visit his parents for the weekend. She was bored and uncomfortable at his parents and didn't want to go. Result: She

went with him. The following weekend they drove to a pottery factory to shop, which was something she wanted to do.

They Are Faithful

Affairs are risky for the marriage relationship. Having an affair is like riding on empty—you never know when it is going to end (run out of gas) and you may be a long way from the marital station when it does. They focus on each other and not on someone outside of their relationship.

They Are Flexible

Heraclitus observed, "Nothing endures but change." Spouses in marriages that last are flexible. Such flexibility becomes particularly important when the office lovers discover that their lives include the rearing of children, the management of their respective careers, and the caring for aging parents. Crisis events in the form of alcoholism, death of parents and unexpected health problems also require adaptation. The need for flexibility never ends.

They Have Strong Egos

A strong marriage has been likened to two pillars on opposite ends supporting a flat marble surface. The stability of the marriage is in reference to the independently strong supports. And the distance they are from each other adds to the stability.

A weak marriage has been likened to two pillars that are placed together in the middle underneath the flat marble surface. The marble block is less stable because the supports underneath aren't independent enough (far enough apart) of each other to hold it up. If spouses aren't their own person, can't make independent decisions, and can't function without each other, they put an enormous burden on the partner who is expected to make all the decisions and to "hold up" the other person.

They Enjoy Sex

Sex has been referred to as the icing on the cake. Sex won't make a good marriage but it can make a good one better. And although good sex between partners won't insure that the partners will stay together, it provides one more reason why they want to.

A good sex life enhances a couple's out-of-bed relationship by giving them good memories of shared physically pleasurable events. A 3,000-year-old inscription on the wall of an Egyptian tomb emphasizes the inherent pleasure in physical contact:

> If I kiss her and her lips are open,

> I am happy even without beer.

And Woody Allen is known for his statement, "I've never had a bad orgasm," which is to say that sex is one of the times it always feels good to interact with your partner.

Intercourse also provides the context for intimate sharing. Many spouses talk before and after intercourse about issues, which require a deep level of intimacy. They are alone in their love flight and relish in the togetherness they share.

They Empathize

There are few people with whom we share a close emotional relationship . . . few with whom we share very private information about the intimate details of our lives. Spouses who go the distance with each other have the capacity to understand and have empathy for what their partner is experiencing. "He understands me," said one wife, "he always has." Such empathy encourages a strong emotional bond between the partners. And it is this emotional bond (not fear of divorce or dread of telling one's parents of a divorce) that partners have for each other that is the real reason why they stay together.

SOME MYTHS ABOUT SPOUSES IN MARRIAGES THAT LAST

Just as there are qualities of relationships that go the distance, there are certain myths about relationships that last.

Myth 1: Spouses in Lasting Relationships Are Always Happy

Perhaps the greatest myth of spouses in stable and loving relationships is that they are always happy. We tend to assume that their marriage is immune from the normal ups and downs in any relationship.

It isn't. Ask any spouse in any marriage how happy he or she is and the answer you get depends on when you ask the person. Their marriage is just like your current or most recent relationship. There have been times when you were so deliriously happy with your partner that you believed the intensity of these feelings would last forever. But there have been other times when you felt less than positive (to say the least) about your partner because of something he or she did, said, or didn't do or say. One woman said that when her partner didn't get her a Valentine's Day card she could have packed his suitcase and thrown him out. "After all," she said, "it wouldn't take much time to drive to the drugstore and invest a little time in thinking about me. And when he let Valentine's Day go by without giving me anything, I didn't want to speak to him for a week."

If we believe that the 60 million plus married couples are continuously happy behind closed doors, we delude ourselves and set an artificial standard of what happy, lasting marriages are all about. Living with someone in an intimate relationship is a complicated experience. Because the needs of each partner cannot always be met at the same time, the chance of unabated happiness over several decades is zero.

Myth 2: Spouses in Lasting Relationships Do Not Have Problems

Related to the absence of continuous happiness is the presence of problems. The fact that individuals love each other and are committed to each other does not mean that they are immune to problems, often serious ones. Few couples avoid sickness, financial worries, and child-rearing issues. How these problems are viewed and dealt with makes the difference between marriages that flourish and those that fall apart.

Myth 3: Spouses in Lasting Relationships Do Not Seek Therapy

Another myth about spouses in marriages that last is that they never thumb through the Yellow Pages in search of a therapist. Spouses in lasting marriages are thought to have problems that are minor, or to have the skills to cope with them without seeking outside help. Nonsense. Spouses who are deeply committed to each other may be more likely to seek marriage therapy rather than muddle through their problems or divorce.

Spouses who seek therapy do not accept certain beliefs that prevent troubled spouses from seeking therapy. One is the belief of naturalism—that either you have it or you don't, and that if you "click" as spouses you certainly don't need help with your life. Another belief is that if you need to see a therapist, your marriage is already in trouble, so a therapist would be of little help. In reality, seeking therapy can be viewed as a sign of strength—the spouses recognize their need to get some fresh ideas/direction rather than continue a downward spiral and divorce.

Myth 4: Spouses in Lasting Relationships Are Rich

The frustrations that we have in reference to money (too little of it!) sometimes lead us to think that if we didn't have money problems, we would not have relationship problems. The extension of that belief is that those who don't have as many difficulties in their relationships have more money than those who do. It is true that money helps—that the divorce rate is lower for those with higher incomes. But to assume that if we had piles of money we would be happy in our marriages is to delude ourselves.

Myth 5: Spouses in Marriages That Last Are Lucky

Finally, we sometimes assume that spouses in marriage that last just lucked into their bliss. They met the right person at the right time, have had no trouble getting jobs they enjoy, and have had no problems of alcoholism, infidelity, and on and on.

In one sense, luck is an element of any lasting relationship. There are too many potential things to go wrong in marriage for an element of good fortune not to be involved. But in another sense, lasting marriages don't just happen by themselves. They are the result of conscientious spouses who care about each other and who struggle to keep each other and their relationship on track.

LESSONS FROM SPOUSES IN MARRIAGES THAT LAST

We can learn at least three things from spouses in marriages that last.

The Characteristics May Vary

Marital success depends on a lot of factors, including spending time together, being committed, communicating, compromising, being flexible, etc. And no marriage reflects all of these characteristics all the time. Prioritizing the relationship and working together to make it a good one is probably what makes the difference.

The Relationship Is the Thing

Second, how the spouses feel about each other and what they do in reference to each other is the ball game. Spending time together, compromising differences, and being empathetic have more to do with insuring a lasting marriage than whether the spouses earn $100,000 a year. The spouses themselves, not the loot or the house or the condo at the beach, are the essence of their relationship.

The Benefits Are Worth the Effort

The emotional satisfaction resulting from being part of a lasting marriage is tremendous. Spouses develop unique shared personal histories. Having lived together for 40 or 50 years, they can view each other in reference to the memories that they have shared and that they are yet to create. "We're all after the same thing," said one spouse, who had been married 48 years. "We want to love someone and be loved. And when you've been able to make it through thick and thin with the same person across time, it gives you a special feeling for your partner and your relationship." Office lovers hope to transition from the workplace to the home place. There is no reason they cannot do so successfully.

CAUTIONS: BEFORE YOU WALK DOWN THE AISLE

Love is a drug that alters our judgment. We see things that aren't there (the partner drinks too much but we say that he is "just having a good time") or don't see things that are very obvious (he only wants to meet at your apartment to have sex). In addition to clearing the love haze, keep in mind some other things before taking that short walk down the aisle.

Run the Clock for Two Years

Don't rush into marriage. Even if your office romance has taken off like a rocket, slow it down. Researchers have found that lovers who know each other for a couple of years before tying the marital knot tend to report happier, more durable marriages.[9] One reason for waiting two years is that the longer you know someone, the more opportunity you have to see the person in a variety of contexts. In addition to seeing the person at the office for six months, take extended trips together and get to know his or her friends. The greater the variety of contexts in which you can experience your partner, the better.

Have a Great Deal in Common

If there is one factor to keep in mind when deciding if you want to marry your office love, it is to ensure that you have a great deal in common. Studies consistently show that the more you have in common (education, social class, religion, age, race, etc.) the more likely you are to be happily married, and to stay married.[10] Similar backgrounds, values, goals, and interests provide a foundation for the development of an intense friendship.

Notice that your closest friends are those with whom you have much in common. If you and your office love are completely different, you might want to run the clock longer than two years before getting married. While love and lust will divert you from the need to be involved with someone with whom you have a lot in common, the need to share common interests will not go away. Pay attention to this issue since it will resurface.

The second author of this book has seen over 1,000 couples in marriage counseling. Not one has ever said, "We have so much in common that we are bored silly." Indeed, these couples are less likely to be in marriage counseling since they are off enjoying a shared activity. "We have nothing in common" is the more frequent comment made by couples in marriage counseling.

Take Parental Approval Seriously

While love is a private matter, marriage is a public event. A relationship that began in the office as private winking, flirting, lunches, and dinners will end up being known by office mates, colleagues, and parents. The approval of your parents is particularly important, as it is associated with subsequent marital happiness.[11] Not only do your parents know you well, they are not blinded by the love you feel for your partner, so their judgment may be more clear.

Of course, the ultimate decision is yours-you can marry your office love whether they like it or not. But give some thought to their opinion of this person as your mate. As an aside, it is rare for parents to disapprove of the mate choice of their son or daughter- only 13 percent do.[12]

End an Abusive Relationship Now

Over four million women in the U.S. are physically harmed by their husbands or intimates.[13] A higher number are emotionally/psychologically abused in terms of their partner slinging insults at them names ("fat," "slut," "stupid") or denigrating them ("you are pathetic and no one else would want you"). Once the abuse in a relationship begins, it escalates. Getting out for many victims is difficult since they profess they are in love, feel unalterably dependent, and don't see a way out. Seeing a counselor to discuss one's escape may be helpful. But ending an abusive office romance is the thing to do.

On-and-Off Relationship

On-and-off office relationships do not bode well for a successful marriage. Such roller-coaster relationships reflect a pattern: an argument reaches a point where the partners can't stand the conflict any longer, they decide not to see each other for a few days, they have a make-up period, and then they repeat the cycle. Before marriage, the partners can easily retreat to their respective homes. After marriage, leaving becomes more difficult. Yet staying in the same house can increase already heightened tensions. If your relationship reflects this on-and-off pattern, consider delaying any plans to marry until you have a sustained period devoid of it. Otherwise, your marriage is likely to repeat your pre-marriage period—and not have a good outcome.

GETTING MARRIED FOR THE WRONG REASON

In the 2009 movie *Up in the Air*, George Clooney plays a character so emotionally detached that he basically lives his lonely life in airports between job assignments. Who captures his interest for making a real connection? Naturally, a woman who doesn't force the issue and appears to accept a casual fling and the fly-by encounter. A female who sees this movie may ask, How could she be so cool and collected about this guy who, if far from romantic is, after all, George Clooney?

In any event, *Up in the Air* illustrates an affair that is office-centric and thereby permits, or tempts, somebody to show only a partial identity.

Office romances are not immune from the partners deciding to wed for the wrong reason. Make sure none of these apply to you.

Status/Money

If your office love is the boss and his or her status or net worth is the primary attraction, beware. Once you get your lover home, you may feel a hole in your heart the size of a grapefruit. In the United States, we marry for love and are taught that mercenary motives are something to be ashamed of. Furthermore, love (in the United States) is the primary quality that sustains relationships. We interviewed office workers who said that they "married the boss" because it was a "good deal," not because it was a "love deal." While these individuals are still married, they lament that staying married for someone to pay the Visa bill has its own cost.

Pregnancy

In spite of knowing how to prevent conception, couples at the office sometimes get pregnant. Peggy of *Mad Men* got pregnant by Pete. While some opt for an abortion (as did Peggy), others may feel pressure to speed up the relationship and the wedding. We encourage you to slow down. Marriages which occur because of an unexpected pregnancy are vulnerable to divorce. The haunting question of the respective spouses is, "Would we have married had there not been a pregnancy?" While some couples would answer "yes" other couples look at each other with an implied "maybe," or a certain "no."

If you are a pregnant office couple, separate the pregnancy from your view of the relationship as loving and nurturing and of the marriage as worthy on its own merits. In effect, keep the relationship on the same clock that was running before the pregnancy occurred. You may decide to get married now. Alternatively, you may continue to develop your relationship. Either outcome is okay.

Pity

Most office romances begin when both partners are in good physical health. And good health usually continues as the relationship develops.

Sometimes, however, one of the partners has a life-altering accident or contracts a progressive disease. The latter happened to Mark, who began to show symptoms of MS (multiple sclerosis) after dating Maria for a year.

Maria faced a dilemma. While she loved Mark, she had an uncle with MS, so she knew the debilitating effect of the disease over time. Indeed, she had begun to pity Mark as he stumbled down the steps and began to slur his words. She reevaluated her decision to marry him. She decided not to continue the relationship, and told him of her decision. As it turned out, Mark had his own hesitancies about continuing the relationship.

A person's changed health status may or may not have a detrimental effect on a couple's relationship (office romance or otherwise). We recommend that partners discuss the new physical changes and how it impacts their thinking about the future. That the couple can talk about such a sensitive issue is a positive comment on their relationship. What they decide to do will vary with the couple—there is no right answer.

Rebound

If your office love is on the rebound from a previous relationship, be cautious. In a study of 1,002 adults, over half (53%) reported that they had become involved in a new relationship while they were on the rebound.[14] When these people were compared with those who had not become involved while on the rebound, the former revealed some negative characteristics, including being love seekers, deceptive, and hedonistic. Being a love seeker meant that the person on the rebound was much more likely to believe in love at first sight. Hence, while your office mate may have shown an instant attraction to you, he or she may also be on the rebound and vulnerable to any new love.

Dishonesty was another quality associated with being on the rebound. Almost three-quarters (72%) of the rebounders reported having been dishonest in a previous relationship (in contrast to only 45 percent who reported having been dishonest who were not on the rebound).

Finally, rebounders were more likely to be hedonistic in regard to sexual values than those who were not on the rebound (73% versus 61%). They also were less likely to use a condom in their sexual encounters. Finding out if your partner is on the rebound is a good idea. If so, run the clock on the relationship to help ensure that this is the person whom you want to marry. If you are on the rebound, give yourself time to recover from your previous relationship before moving forward in a marriage.

Escape

While lovers enjoy seeing each other, having lunch, etc., at the workplace, they may come from and return to dealing with people from whom they want to escape. Such was the case of Jim and Ruth—he was living with his alcoholic parents who fought all the time; she was living with a roommate who "smoked all the time and had her drunken boyfriends over." Both wanted to escape their home lives and get married.

Lovers who are motivated more by leaving an aversive situation than by being drawn to each other may discover that they made a mistake. In retrospect, they may feel that they were in such a hurry to leave that they did not adequately explore their own relationship. Without love, common interests, and goals, lovers can end up worse off than in the situations from which they came. If you are in a love relationship with someone at work and are considering marriage, make sure that you are motivated more by wanting to be *with* your partner than wanting to escape *from* a negative situation.

As we close this chapter, we emphasize that office lovers end up in good marriages when they have the personal and relationship qualities that are true of happy and durable relationships. Office loves are exciting, but taking them on the marital trip is another matter. By giving their relationship time to cook (a couple of years), and ensuring that interests and values are shared, they may have the beginning of a wonderful life together.

THE PLUSES AND MINUSES OF BEING SPOUSES AT THE OFFICE[15]

Dr. Marie McIntyre is a workplace psychologist in Georgia and the author of *Secrets to Winning at Office Politics*. She identifies how spouses benefit and what they might look out for when they work for the same company.

> I've found that many workplace couples do remain with the same company, especially if they work in different areas. Sharing an employer has a number of benefits, ranging from the dual commute to simply understanding more about your spouse's life. When your wife comes home complaining about her ditzy boss, you may actually know what she's talking about!

On the other hand, there are risks, including the danger of losing both jobs if the business hits a rough patch. And couples have to be sure that discussion of office politics doesn't dominate their domestic conversations. There is definitely some benefit to having an escape from work at home, so office couples often have to establish guidelines about when to turn off the office talk.

When one of the spouses of a workplace couple leaves for greener (or at least different) pastures, challenges can arise if the person goes to work for a competitor of their spouse's company. Bosses can become wary of couples sharing proprietary information, and it can be difficult to constantly screen what you are telling your spouse. . . . kind of like working for the CIA.

Another issue is keeping your spouse and work roles separate. If the partners interact frequently in the course of their work, the key is learning to clearly separate the work relationship from the personal relationship. At home, you are a spouse. At work, you are a colleague. And at work you do not engage in spouse behavior. No affectionate touches, private jokes, whispered confidences, and so forth. You want to treat your spouse just as you do your other colleagues—friendly, polite, respectful, considerate, helpful, etc.

And it goes without saying that you do NOT bring your arguments and disagreements to the office. Even if you're furious, you have to be able to slip into colleague behavior at work. Your boss and your coworkers do not need to be burdened with your domestic disputes. Or even hear about them. Yes, this can get a bit schizophrenic. And people who can't pull it off should not continue to work in the same place.

So what specifically should individuals think about before marrying someone at the office? All of the above, of course. But also, before marrying a coworker, people need to be sure that they know the "real" person. When you've worked with someone for a long time, it's easy to think that you really know them. But at the office, all you see is their work personality, which is a very limited view. So before settling down with someone, be sure that you've spent enough time getting to know all aspects of their character. People who marry colleagues too hastily sometimes encounter unpleasant and unexpected surprises behind the "work mask." Indeed, they need to remember that the office is a social context/little world of its own, where people share goals and frustrations and successes and failures.

FUTURE EXPECTATIONS—CAREER OR TRADITIONAL WIFE?

In deciding to marry someone you fell in love with at the office, you want to look ahead and discuss future job/career/family plans. When a career man is no longer in the role (either he was fired, or he has decided to leave the fast track to raise honeybees or be a whitewater guide for a living), his role change will require his partner to adjust accordingly. If the woman requires that her man be "Mr. Career" and he wants to raise bees, the partners may split. Alternatively, she may delight in his role change. If they have children they may both benefit from his being Mr. Mom. Take for example the couple where she is the pediatrician and he is the stay-at-home dad with their two children.

Alternatively, suppose the woman at the office is "Ms. Career," but after marriage she decides she has had enough and wants to stay home and care for the children. Can her partner adapt as she morphs into mommy? Women who meet their husbands when both are fully employed and career-oriented need to be aware that their partners and they themselves may *change*. Considering the possibilities and discussing them ahead of time is exactly what the couple should do. Indeed, does he expect you to continue your money-making career (which means a two-income family) or take after his mother, the consummate homemaker (which means he will be the happy provider)?

And what are his expectations in regard to child care when children arrive (and by the way, does he want any)? If you remain a significant breadwinner, how will he feel about taking the child to daycare every morning? Or, will he say that daycare is so expensive that you might as well stay home? Or will he support you for having earned a master's degree and wanting to keep you hand in your career? These are conversations you must have. It will be an eye-opening talk leading to, optimally, two people saying they will try this or that and work it out, with some tentative 2-, 5- and 10-year plans.

My (Jane, first author) daughter-in-law and her two older sisters were raised in a family where girls were encouraged to have a career and to excel. In the course of five years, all three had married and had had a child. The middle sister, who has two boys, considers herself fully occupied staying at home with her children; her husband is happy with this decision but open to her returning to her career later. The older sister and her husband met when both had demanding careers in Washington, D.C. She has enjoyed staying home with her daughter, but now that the child is entering first grade, she plans to reenter the job force.

As for my daughter-in-law, she took a six-month maternity leave and returned to work on a part-time basis, so that the baby was in day care three full days a week. The couple negotiated all of this, which is tricky territory. "I can do it all ... sometime," said my daughter-in-law. Another mother told me, *"You can do it all if you will expand your time horizons. In other words, I'm 30 and I'm going to work for about 35 more years. I'm not driven to be executive director because I value my personal life too much and this arrangement my family's needs at this stage. If I had a rock star job it might be harder; but my friend, who has her ideal job, into which she has poured all of herself, says she has other competing priorities now. For me, part-time work and being at home part-time feels exactly right. Burton [her husband] used to say the same thing over the months we discussed it 'It's all up to you' and I knew he meant it . . . You have to have someone whose passion is you and the baby. Because he and I are theoretically and practically in accord, it was okay when we had our baby and I realized, 'I'm not as driven as I thought.'"*

Each partner comes with expectations relating to earnings, child rearing, and sharing daily tasks, which need to be understood and in synch. There is no clear-cut solution. The issues often need to be revisited depending on the stage of the family life cycle.

12

Trade Secrets of the Ultimate Office Romance

Our greatest fear in life is not that it will end but that it will never begin.
J. H. Newman

Love is wonderful wherever you find it. And more than just a few are finding it at the office. Forty percent of the 8,038 fulltime employed, nongovernment workers reported that they had dated someone at the office.[1] But since love has the capacity to be as devastating as it is wonderful, in this chapter we review some trade secrets for the ultimate office romance identified by those whom we interviewed.

MEET YOUR OFFICE LOVE ON OR OFF THE CLOCK

In the study referred to above, 88 percent met on the job.[2] One of the office workers we interviewed said:

> When we were first assigned to work on a project together, he was the last person I wanted from the office pool, he was the scrawny technical guy. But he turned out to be a polite, respectful, egalitarian, hard-working man whom I looked forward to seeing when I came to work. I never wanted the day to end at 5:00. He simply "grew" on me.

About 20 percent of office workers in this survey reported having had more than one office love.

Twelve percent reported that they had run into each other away from the office, 10 percent at happy hour and 10 percent at lunch.[3] At these co- or extracurricular events, the employees felt free to approach and engage the person face-to-face. These are also more relaxing contexts. Not only has the person left the stress of the job back at the office, but the office party/happy hour also allows people to have a drink or two, kick back, and become more social. Some reported that they enjoyed their office mate in these contexts for weeks, maybe months, before they became involved and began to have their own happy hour or lunch.

USE THE OFFICE TO PLAY AFTER HOURS? (SOME DO!)

While the demands of the job will put a damper on being with/interacting with one's office love, these demands will not stop it. The 8,000 plus respondents in the CareerBuilder.com survey gave examples of "some of the most romantic things" they did on site (in the office/at the workplace). These included dancing to the elevator music in the hallway, having a late-night picnic with candles after everyone had left, and having a drink together on the roof of the building. Our interviewees also told us of sex on the desk, the office couch, the floor, etc. In the main, as the office closed for the day, the "open for romance" sign suddenly appeared. In effect, participants spoke of enjoying at/in their jobs more because they were together all day, and to boot, sometimes using the office as a private playground after hours.

ENJOY THE LOVE RIDE

The opening quote for this chapter emphasizes that love is the ultimate life experience. Whether you find love at the office or online, it provides the magical high. Our respondents who had had office lovers revealed that working at the same place provided the ideal context for a romantic relationship: they could see each other every work day and they loved every minute of it.

DELAY THE SEX

As we mention in Chapter 13, the research on 'When the Relationship Becomes Sexual" confirms that both parties and their relationship have a great deal to gain by delaying the sex. A quick and certain end to the office romance is to introduce sex too early into the relationship. What is "too early"? Clearly, only the lovers can decided what is best for them, but one-third of the 429 respondents in one study reported that they regretted having had sex "too soon."[4] This was more the case for women than for men (35 versus 27 percent).[5] The take-home message is to enjoy the teasing, slow sensual sexual build-up over months of tacit flirting in the office, letting the sexual interest rise to a slow boil before having your first cup. A mere 3 percent of 429 respondents said that they had their first intercourse "too late."[6] The trade secret to the ultimate office romance is to *slow down and wait before you include sex in your relationship!*

DELAY SAYING "I LOVE YOU"

Just as advisable as delaying the first sex (intercourse) experience, is delaying the declaration of one's love. In the study of 429 respondents mentioned above, over one-quarter (26%) reported that they regretted saying "I love you" "too soon"[7] and less than 4 percent (3.9%) reported that they regretted saying it "too late."[8] The problem with expressing your love too soon is that your partner may not feel the same way. The result is a feeling of obligation and a prolonged silence followed by a weak "Yes . . . . I love you too," which translates to "You blew it . . . why did you have to bring that up the L word now?" The trade secret is to wait until your partner tells you that he or she loves you . . . saving you from jeopardizing the relationship in that way.

DECIDE NEVER TO BE PHYSICAL AT THE OFFICE

While you may be pulsating with desire to be physical with your new love, behave yourself. Do not touch, hug, caress, or kiss at the office. You are on company time. Demonstrative behavior and all physical gestures should occur only on your own time. What about a covert kiss in the copy room? You can probably get away with it once—28 percent of the 774 respondents in our Internet Office Romance Survey said that they had; however, the danger is that not being caught will reinforce the behavior. That touch to the wrist or flounce of the hair will escalate to a kiss to virtual foreplay once the match is struck. The risk of being caught will then increase by leaps and bounds. Although 67 out of 5,000 respondents in an updated CareerBuilders.com office romance study said that their relationship was not a secret to people they worked with,[9] don't flaunt it. Your first priority is your job.

KEEP YOUR OFFICE LOVE PROFESSIONAL IN THE OFFICE

Not being physical with your lover in the office is an example of keeping your relationship professional when at the office. This translates into not always sitting together at employee meetings, lunching with fellow employees rather than exclusively with each other, voting as an individual not as a couple, disagreeing openly when an issue is being discussed at an employee meeting, and, need we mention, not sending each other cards, flowers, balloons, and such. Keeping your relationship professional removes it from being an issue in the department that bosses or fellow employees have to contend with. For example, one couple that worked in the same firm never insisted that they be sent on the same assignment or travel together. This opened up a slot for other members to work with one or the other, such as on a project or business trip. The trade secret is to conduct your love relationship in the office as though there isn't one.

AVOID OFFICE E-MAILS/TEXTING

While occasional e-mails to each other are appropriate (such as,"What time are you leaving work today?") constant electronic communication with each other is a no-no. Not only is this amateurish, but it provides a trail should your boss or his want to fire you for spending your day e-mailing and texting each other. Refrain.

DO YOUR JOB

Without a doubt, your 9-to-5 focus should always be on the work you are paid to do. The corporation may benefit from your relationship since they have two good workers who are likely to stay with the firm (eliminating costly rehiring). Similarly, you and your partner may benefit from being able to ride to work together, have an occasional lunch together, and have a shared understanding of your workday. However, this and the good cheer (not ebullience) you display is the extent to which your relationship should impact the workplace. Doing your job will remove the relationship from being an issue to your respective bosses.

ACCEPT THAT YOUR OFFICE ROMANCE DOESN'T HAVE
TO END IN MARRIAGE

In the CareerBuilder. Com survey, almost one-third (32%) of those who had office romances reported that they ended in marriage.[10] This means that the majority of the office romances did *not* end in marriage. If you keep your expectations for the future of your relationship realistic, the office romance is likely to have a positive outcome regardless of whether you marry. Doubtless, the fact that you don't get married can be as positive an outcome as if you do.

Office romances do not end in marriage for the same reasons that adult relationships generally end—there is somebody else, a lack of chemistry, differences too great to bridge, or one person moves away. One example of having great differences is a man from India who was expected to marry someone from his own culture and religion. The fact that the couple had a great love and sex life could not be trumped by their respective backgrounds. He ended up leaving the firm to go back to India. She was heartbroken, but would have felt that way whether they were in the same office or not.

Having to see someone with whom you have just ended a relationship with can be difficult. The second author sat next to a colleague in a faculty meeting once who whimpered throughout the meeting. She had just broken up with another faculty member who happened to be sitting on the other side of the table. Sometimes the pain is so great that the person will quit or transfer. In this case, she left. She is not alone. Nine percent of the respondents in our Internet survey reported that they looked back on their office romance with regret. In the CareerBuilder.com survey, of those who became involved in an office romance, 5 percent reported that they left their job due to the office romance.[11]

AVOID AN STI/DISCOVERING A LOVER'S PAST
AND REVEALING YOUR OWN

Having the ultimate office romance means avoiding contracting a sexually transmissible disease (now known as an STI; this was formerly known as a sexually transmitted disease, or STD). Because of the fear of HIV infection and other STIs, it is prudent to know the details of each other's previous sex life, including how many partners he or she has had sex with and in what contexts (stable relationships or hooking up).

Naturally, talking about a partner's previous sex life is a touchy subject. And lovers lie to each other. Almost one in four (23.9%) of 1,319 reported having lied to a partner about their previous number of sexual partners.[12] Even in "monogamous" relationships, there is considerable lying. In one study of 1,341 college students, 27.2 percent of the males and 19.8 percent of the females reported having oral, vaginal, or anal sex outside of a relationship that their partner considered monogamous. People most likely to cheat in these "monogamous" relationships were men over the age of 20, those who were binge drinkers, and those who reported that they were "nonreligious." [13] Hence, while trying to find out the sexual history of your office lover is a good idea, good luck on getting a straight answer! And even if you feel that you and your office lover are exclusive, some studies reveal this may not be the case.

BE TRANSPARENT—LET YOUR EMPLOYER KNOW WHAT IS GOING ON[14]

According to Lois Frankel, Ph.D., president of Corporate Coaching International, and author of *Nice Girls Don't Get the Corner Office*, office romances involve "a unique situation that requires unique people to pull it off seamlessly." She tells her executive clients (not married, naturally) who start up an office romance to be direct and clear in their communications with each other and their employer—"This will always serve you well."

What gets people in the most trouble is when it looks like you're trying to hide something. The most important thing is transparency—to be open about what you are doing. If you are about to date someone in the office, read the company policy and inform the boss and HR if that is the policy. If you have nothing to hide, you have nothing to hide.

You would naturally bring the person you are seeing to events or invite them to your home with friends. And when you go to HR, you can say, "I'm delighted. I'm dating someone in the ABC department." It sounds grown-up! You might not do this after the first date, in case the relationship doesn't work out, but when it's clear that the relationship will be ongoing, do this so no one is blindsided.

Another consideration for a successful office romance identified by Dr. Frankel is that the lovers must be aware that issues can become complicated. For example, one of her clients was up for a promotion she deserved, but had recently moved in with someone senior to her in the company. When her promotion was reviewed, those tenured in the company asked, "Can she be trusted?" and "Does she really need this job?" *A woman has to be prepared for the repercussions. As long as she was living with this senior guy, her career was in jeopardy of being eclipsed.*

Alternatively, if a woman has a high-level position, say a senior vice-president, and she is dating a manager, her judgment may be questioned. And if it's a reporting relationship, there can be trouble when the relationship goes south, whether the person in the junior position is a man or woman. There is always the potential for a sexual harassment claim—"the only reason I went out with my boss was that I thought my job was in jeopardy if I didn't" will be the script of the junior person who got dumped.

13

When the Office Romance Becomes Sexual

You look as though you are waiting to be asked.

Office Pick-Up Line

Given that almost 40 percent (37%) of 5,231 employees in the CareerBuilder.com survey acknowledged that they had dated someone at the office, we can reasonably assume that some of these relationships involved sex.[1] One-quarter of the respondents in our Internet survey stated that their office fling had become sexual.

Women inevitably confront the issues of sex and romance in the workplace. Most are reluctant to risk ruining their jobs by having trysts with the guys. While the reason for caution about office sex might have been virginity in years past, today it is because people value their jobs. The sexual activity on the job seems to come later, when older professional women are trying out potential partners. At that point, they are fairly sexually experienced as they go into their first office affair.

Like a match, sex ignites and brings life, light, and warmth; it also burns. While a level of sexual tension in the workplace can make people smile and feel lighthearted, when two people pair off as lovers, everybody but them stands outside looking in. In Mozart's opera *The Marriage of Figaro*, the music changes from a cheery jig to a complex duet when the Count's two servants try to change their status from popular flirts to an exclusive relationship (fiancés). As soon as people begin to find out, the music becomes both more vivid and more urgent, with quick tempos and dark notes.

Sex is not a tranquilizer, but a stimulant. An established couple has sex for various reasons and when they're in different moods—to reconnect or play, in a state of desire or aglow with love—but a sexual relationship that occurs in the workplace is not going to be relaxed until it is taken *out* of the workplace. People who are very ambitious have to deny their pleasure and their impulse to give or receive affection when they are on the job. They focus and gain work momentum. Interviews that Jane did for Executive Health Examiners revealed that since the executives were exhausted from constant conferences, if they wanted to relax, they were more likely to play golf than cozy up to an attractive woman in the work environment. Moreover, studies in the late 1970s, in which executives were often depicted as studs, found, contrarily, that executives who made it to the top tended to have supportive spouses and stable family units. If the top guns had hidden lives they were very well hidden; only a small minority had a "double life" that made lurid news.[2]

Sex belongs off-premises. Those who have sex on the job do so with great care. A female attorney who looks at conservation easements recalled when her staff was ordered into the field to prospect potential tracts of land:

> I thought I was immune to infatuation, but the assignment had complicated issues. A co-worker and I had intense talks around the campfire, and started falling in love. Awash with desire one night, deep in the woods, I crawled into his tent. At each step of lovemaking he asked, "Are you sure?" I was sure! But we never repeated it. I spoke in such glowing terms of the trip that my boss wanted to see for himself. He organized another trip a month later for a group of us over the same terrain. I went with trepidation, but the co-worker and I just gave each other scorching looks: we were not going to risk our professional credibility for "summer love."

Armies have dealt with the trouble that fraternization stirs up for millennia. "Trouble brews when it's between two people of different ranks," said retired General Walter Lippincott, a law professor and former counsel for the Coast Guard.[3] He continued:

> Military fraternization law and policy applies to commissioned and warrant officers, who are the corporate officers of the military services. Fraternization limits the familiarity between officers and enlisted service members. The specific conduct prohibited is not identified in the law, but it clearly does not limit its prohibitions to improper sexual relations. It is any conduct that is prejudicial to good order, discrediting to the

military services and to enforcing good discipline among the services. Examples of prohibited fraternization activities are dating and sexual relations between officers and enlisted members, commercial activities like renting and sale of property, and gambling by military members of different ranks.

SINGLE AND AMBITIOUS

In the classic movie, *All about Eve*, Bette Davis hands center stage over to a younger and more ambitious woman because she realizes she wants to settle down with a good guy. She tells her best friend: "Funny business, a woman's career. The things you drop on the way up the ladder so you can move faster, you forget you'll need them again when you get back to being a woman."

Today's woman of 20 to 30 is likely to be thinking school and career first, then marriage and family. When a woman with a successful career encounters an eligible and desirable man through work, it can often be the next item on her agenda. Priscilla's work decorum at the transportation company was flawless; she was an irreproachable member of the corps of people who made decisions and ran the company. *I didn't manipulate or seduce Aaron*, she said, *but when he divorced I set out to get him with all my pistons firing. I made the move to have sex by inviting myself to his apartment the first time we went out. I admired his performance on the job, and I was sure he'd be a wonderful partner in bed. I knew so much about him, and it was all good. He respected me. I wasn't going to hold back on sex anymore than I do in other aspects of my life.*

Other women echoed this idea: that the "third-date rule" had nothing to do with when their relationship with a workmate would became sexual. The sexual encounter was usually preceded by a long getting-to-know-you period; once they actually dated, they had sex right away. Hence, one advantage of having sex with someone you meet at the office is that you have time to develop a relationship with him.

THE WORKPLACE THAT SPARKLES

"In your dreams!" winked and whispered an agent going to the break room, when a guy looked up from his desk and blew her a kiss. *Isn't this risky behavior, I thought, when I began working as part of their company.*

Audra was speaking of a company where the element of liveliness in male-female relationships was present in spades. *The funny thing was that away from work, they were all in a relationship with somebody—either married or involved. But at work, a lot of the workers acted like lovers. They had so much fun—at lunch and sitting on each other's desks. I'd worked for that company for a year when I was invited to celebrate the design firm's big new contract abroad. They were drinking champagne and carrying on as usual, only with their children and spouses in the mix. The owners were a couple who had met as architects. They adored each other, and that energy lit everybody up. When I finished college, my sister warned me that not all workplaces functioned like this.*

WHERE SEX OCCURS

As noted at the beginning of this chapter, sex on the job is not unusual. Midge thought about being a showgirl and went to Vegas. However, she liked working for a florist so much that she stayed with that. She spoke about how she fell in love with a co-worker. *We weren't supervised. We loved the business and our boss was a wonderful, crazy character talented up the kazoo. When Paolo was hired, I trained him. It's typical to come into the flower business from some unrelated background—Paolo had played on a national soccer team in South America. I saw the beautiful, natural skill he had with the flowers, and that he wasn't conceited or two-faced. I was crazy about him but never let on. Then we did these huge arrangements for a hotel wedding. The afternoon before the wedding, we began kissing like mad behind the curtains during the rehearsal. I remember thinking, "I want you now, but I don't want you to think I'm a slut." Then I realized that we had been working together sometimes 12 hours a day and often at night, and there was no way that he would think badly of me. You have to have two things for a good relationship—great sex and great trust. We had both.*

TALKING ABOUT THE SEX TO OTHERS?

Almost 30 percent of the respondents in our Internet survey reported that they told someone of their office romance. Lovers suspect that if they tell a soul—and the chances are one of them will disclose there is something going on—that the gossip may begin. Cass works for a fine ceramics company as a liaison to their Spanish and Italian factories. She was warned when she took the job not to fraternize, although there was no written company policy. Sure she could keep a secret, Cass and the son of the head of the Spanish firm started a passionate relationship. The father invited her to lunch and raised it diplomatically.

"He said, 'Where do you want to be in 10 years?' I said, 'What do you mean, sir?' He said, 'Because you are sleeping with my youngest son.' "I said, 'I know he's a playboy, but I am crazy about your son. We're not hurting anybody—it's our business —but how did you find out?' He looked at me with his long Spanish face and the look of ancient knowledge and said, "Three ways, Cassandra. Your eyes they sparkle, your cheeks they glow, and you don't walk, you float.' "

While the lovers' behavior may give them away, it could be that one of the two new lovers may want to show the other off as a prize. This can cause discomfort for the more discreet one. The couple must decide what gradations of public behavior they endorse. In general, the fewer who know the better ... And who wants to be a prize?

THE DAY AFTER

In the long-running TV comedy series *The Office*, there are plot lines involving romance—expressed and unspoken desires between co-workers—as well as hilarity in one episode called "Back from Vacation," where the male head of the office goes to Jamaica with his female superior, and later e-mails a nude photo of her to the whole office by mistake. The moral, of course, is that romance can readily simmer with the people you work with/spend eight hours a day with (more than anyone else), but you have to face them "tomorrow."

CONSEQUENCES OF INTERCOURSE

In one study, 163 unmarried individuals who were involved in a relationship were asked "What effect has having intercourse had on your relationship?" Sixty-three percent reported "no change," while 30 percent reported that sex "improved the relationship."[4] In another study that looked at the effects of various levels of sexual intimacy (from kissing to intercourse) on relationship commitment, the "milder, but more affectionate, behaviors of holding hands and kissing seemed to be more important indicators of couples' commitment than the more intense behaviors of fondling and sexual intercourse."[5] Hence, having intercourse did not seem to move the relationship toward more commitment.

Women have lost control of courtship. Some of them are regaining it. They have lost control by having casual sex. If all they want is casual sex, the status quo of premarital sex is fine. You can learn a lot about a person by connecting intimately. I (Jane, co-author) have long noted, ruefully, that the best way to learn a foreign language is to have a love affair with a native speaker, and I recommend that without reservation to a professional spy. However, most women do not want to have casual sex. Praise Venus, we are looking for love and commitment. That means that if we are having casual sex as young women, we must either feel that it will roll off our backs (rarely true), or that we can gain some knowledge from the bite of this particular apple.

However, the only knowledge that I see women gaining from casual sex is suffering and pain, with the result that they use up seasons of their lives and a lot of energy to cope with breakups; had they loved and had romance without going to bed with the congenial or attractive fellow, wouldn't the suffering have been far less? Wouldn't they have been able to move on to a new, more promising relationship more easily?

If you are very drawn to each other at the office, and you think there is potential, and you start dating, what is the drive that a woman feels? Since the office is anti-intimacy, naturally we exchange feelings and private experiences and feel a physical urge/urgency. The main thing that is happening is that we women think there will be an increase in intimacy when we sleep with the man; in fact, men are more biologically constituted, and the opening of their hearts (and minds—being willing to share their feelings and thought) does not come with sex. Only sex comes with sex!

But if the relationship breaks up, women get hurt afterwards. They feel that they have shared something of themselves, something precious. They have let themselves be vulnerable. To the men, it felt good, and that was that. Vulnerability is something that we learn at school and at work to deny and put up a barricade against. The women interviewed spoke of relationships with co-workers that were very "hot" (because the lid was off on the sex drive) but "went nowhere" and ended with a whimper or thud because the man "only wanted sex." Real intimacy includes trusting that you can be vulnerable, honest and your multifaceted unique self. And that is not a precondition of sex! Why not start with and keep your drawers on instead of having to become strong to face the mess that results from sex before emotional intimacy?

Here's a scenario recommended by many of the women we interviewed:

> You observe the person in a context in which his personality is made gradually known to you, you have co-workers who weigh in with their impression of him and whether you and he are going to be compatible,

you are not going to be seduced and abandoned if he values his job, and so forth. Most importantly, you are not under pressure to sleep with him because the workplace offers a sort of shield, a delay factor, and not a stop sign, but a caution-go slow sign.

Why does a woman need to stay a little detached and not jump into a sexual relationship headfirst? Because of STIs, because serious break-ups can be like driving a car along on a beautiful day and singing along with the radio and then landing in a ditch. So, keep it all "correct" at the workplace for a longer time; try to lead not the "double" life of sleeping with the guy in the next cubicle and sneaking in like culprits the next morning, but a "single" life of courtship where you get acquainted as human beings, establish a level of trust, and see whether you and he have the same goals before you take it to the next level. From what I [Jane] see of younger women, the overriding issue may be acknowledging that they want commitment rather than to sleep with a series of guys so they feel battle-scarred by age 25 or 30 or 35.

It's like being checkmated if, as a woman, you become the one he sleeps with, when during the workday you and he have to mind your Ps and Qs. The situation is rife for misunderstandings: Am I liked, loved, wanted . . . is there a future?

THE MEANING OF SEX FOR MEN AND WOMEN

In a study of 99 never-married adults, men said that they were much more likely than women were to have intercourse with someone they had known for three hours, to have intercourse with someone they did not love, and to have intercourse with someone with whom they did not have a good relationship.[6]

This is where the gender factor has changed very little. The interest of the man at the office to have sexual intercourse does not mean that he has an emotional interest in the woman, and she should not inter-pret such willingness as an interest in her or the future of the relation-ship. From his point of view it is all about sex, not the "relationship."

Women in the same study declared just the opposite. Having inter-course was a reflection that the woman had affectionate feelings for the partner and would be interested in a continuation of the relationship.[7]

Moreover, women need more reassurance as the relationship becomes sexual. One woman we interviewed said that *I operated at work in a self-induced panic over whether we would have sex that night, or not until the weekend, and whether I should worry that he didn't seem fazed.*

Nevertheless, having sex right there in the workplace seems to be something that some women remember with a chuckle and glee; they feel that they were so gutsy—as though this was a zany accomplishment for them, more than proof of irresistible lust.

The biggest difference between men and women is that women obsess about their relationships. Carol Smith, senior vice president for the Elle Group, observed that "female bosses tend to be better managers, better advisers, mentors, rational thinkers . . . but men are definitely better on the 'whatever' side. Things tend to roll off their back. We women take things very personally. We're constantly playing things over in our head—'What did that mean when they said that?'— when they mean nothing."[8]

Men believe the myth that women talk about male physical prowess— the size of their penis, or how many minutes the sexual act lasted. But women do not speak so; rather, they speak of the myriad facets of the relationship. Men do not relate to this. So, once women have sex with them in the office, they are very into it while the men just feel they "got lucky."

But sometimes the sex and relationship go nowhere. One woman said:

> There was one mental health worker who I was interested in. He clearly felt the same way. After years of flirting, and my divorce somewhere in the middle, we dated for about five months. I needed to date him to learn that he was not for me. I have no regrets. He was very tall and beautifully built. He treated me really well, and always planned interesting things for us to do; for instance he took me out on his boat a lot, and I started water-skiing because of him. Ultimately, after battling with myself over why I wasn't enjoying him, briefly believing that it was because he was actually good for me, I finally concluded that he bored me, in spite of all the entertaining.

DARING EXPLOITS

Sex on the premises (evening, weekends, or behind closed doors), relayed by people who had been single when they indulged in them, had a transgressive quality, even though the two who conjugated were single. They spoke of literally wanting to be bad, or wanting to show the other person how bold they were, or that during that period of their life, it was gratifying to be very playful or teasing, e.g., on the rebound.

The top floor of their company was the sandcastle for Derrick, an accountant, and Jeanne, an administrator. *I am the cautious oldest of four children, said Derrick, so Jeannie, the typical mischievous youngest, led us. However, I followed with gusto. We had sex mostly in my office, because the door locks, but in the evening we tried out new positions in new places in and around the building. I told her I'd marry her, but she said that it would spoil the feeling of being wicked if we did the proper thing. Neither of us was hurt. She took a job teaching English in China at the end of that year. In retrospect, I see that she choreographed the affair to bolster her sense of independence before she left.*

Annette, at a law firm for a summer job, said of her office affair with a lawyer:

> The love of my life was actually at the South Pole working as a scientist, and I thought, "This may be my only chance to see what it's like to have sex with another man. Roy was like a vertical element in a horizontal painting—this magnificent exotic person to get to know. He taught me sexual technique and I suppose he became more fluent in English with me. We didn't know any of the same people outside of work. Nobody at work noticed. When we ended it—I was going off to law school in another city and Hans was coming back from the South Pole, we hugged and promised to stay friends.

The office romance usually takes a more serious course. Once the erotic urge is unleashed, emotions run high and unexpected. *From the time we began seeing each other, said Jerri, I was exquisitely wrought up. I came to work the day after we slept together and felt as though I was on the rolling deck of a boat in a stormy sea. I couldn't do my work at the museum, which was quite easy. However, I had to be careful. I couldn't look at him anymore when he came in the room. I felt my work ethic was compromised. We are still dating, by now I work at a gallery. I had to quit my job at the museum.*

It is clear that the outcome of having sex with a co-worker varies. For some, it will be a positive shared memory of a one-time event. For others, sex will be the crowning of an already growing friendship that moves the relationship forward. And for still others, it will start a negative spiral that results in one or both quitting and moving on. In our Internet survey, 9 percent reported that the result of their becoming involved with someone at work was negative.

The take-home message is to be cautious and deliberate in deciding to include sex as part of your relationship. By doing so, you increase the chance of a positive outcome. One fact is certain: when intercourse is delayed, the stability of the relationship is stronger. In a national study of adults aged 15 to 59, 50 percent of couples who waited more than a year after their first meeting to have sexual intercourse ended up getting married; only 10 percent of couples who had sex within the first month of meeting married. [9]

THE MILITARY AS THE OFFICE

Major General Anthony Cucolo, commander of troops in northern Iraq, made it clear that his female soldiers who got pregnant and the fellow soldier who impregnated her could be court-martialed. Hence, while the Army-wide policy was to send a pregnant soldier home, division commanders such as General Cucolo had the authority to impose their own sanctions.[10]

IF YOU WANT MORE THAN SEX

If you want a relationship that lasts past Saturday night, some suggestions include:

It is fine for the woman to tell the man that she loves him and wants him, and if he doesn't feel the same way, and they can't work it out, that she is moving on. She should be gentle, loving, and polite when she says this, not angry and demanding.

Alternatively, put the "L" word under lock and key in the early stages of the relationship. Whisper it only to your dog or cat until you are more sure of him. Then when you do speak of love, it isn't a "throwaway" sort of compliment, but a declaration that asks for a similar, return expression of feeling (and not at once when you spring it on him). Because once you unlock it, you want to have him declare something in the love vocabulary, too.

Don't kowtow, assert. Wear citrus-based perfume if he likes rose, wear jeans if he likes you only in heels and a skirt. The workplace may be where people have to conform, but don't carry that over to your private world.

Don't let a man lie either to himself or to you that everything's fine just because you smile at each other in the hall.

Be fair to an ex-wife, as you and she may have to cooperate some day over driving the kids to soccer practice. What she says about you is neither here nor there; putting you down is par for the course.

If he likes to see you at set intervals that are convenient to him, relegating you to, say, noonsies and Sunday night (if there's no big ball game) explain what you prefer. In the first place, you're accepting crumbs; in the second place, the female libido wells up when we are courted and appreciated, and being in a state of abandonment and desire cannot be fit into his weekly schedule. Meanwhile, do not heed promises such as "I'll never abandon you," because a guy thinks a woman forces him to use such words, generally.

Weave yourself into his life with his friends, particularly old friends, and see if his conduct measures up to what attracted you at work in the first place.

You may be single-mindedly in love. Nevertheless, until you are engaged, you can flirt with another co-worker at lunch.

Martine and Ted met at a sporting goods store where they both worked. He sold boats and she sold clothing. *Normally I'm conservative and shy, but we went to a boat show, it was late, after drinks at dinner, and Ted and I joked about fooling around in one of the boats. We didn't, but the next morning we sat next to each other to hear a speaker and I had to clutch my right hand so I wouldn't reach out to him as he sat next to me. That's how it started—sheer sexual desire—and that's how it evolved. But Ted was serious about being a parent: it was central to his identity (which I admired), and I tried to be understanding when he spent more time arguing with his ex than doing things with me.*

But Martine began to worry that she was being pushed into an unconventional status when she wanted a traditional one. She was right to worry. A year later Ted was talking about marriage as "Martine's issue." He felt happy with things as they were. Meanwhile, Martine had become sick of being introduced as "Ted's girlfriend—they both work for . . . " She gave him a six-month ultimatum to shape up or ship out. *He said he couldn't be with anybody else. I covered my ears when he whined, and a week after we stopped seeing each other he proposed.*

A man sees you waiting, and thinks you wait patiently. Furthermore, his first image of you was at the workplace. If you lose your composure now, with him, you are out of control. If you ask for more of his life, and show need, you are controlling . . . Is this the same woman who seemed so together and smart?

According to Gail, who met her husband working in the Department of Commerce in Washington, D.C.:

> To make a guy who doesn't meet your needs into one who does, you
> have to be prepared to give him an ultimatum (and not to cry wolf).

Unless a man is going to lose you, he thinks "She'll be there at the office the next day" and doesn't know what he has.

Ted didn't want Martine taken away from him, but you may have to take action for a man you work with to see this. You may be in his blind spot. For him to understand that your fuse will end and you'll burn out if you aren't nourished by the eternal kind of love, you have to introduce some brinkmanship—at a sweet moment, naturally, and not overreacting if you don't like what he says. Give the prospective person time.

14

Eight Stories of Office Romance

I went to an employee orientation picnic alone and walked a woman back to her car. We ended up getting married and now have three kids. You never know . . .

A medical student

The real life stories to follow illustrate how love and work intersect and the lives/relationships that unfold as a result.

TWO ATTORNEYS

Priscilla was hired into the large law firm where Tim already worked. She was an attorney who came from another firm, and Tim and she met at a welcome party for new attorneys. Priscilla, fair and willowy with a dancer's poise and composure, was a few years older than Tim and slightly senior to him in position. Tim, solid and athletic, was the kind of popular person people want to have a beer with, but had a keen intelligence and an Ivy League sheen. Tim went to the party feeling curious because they had hired someone senior to him in his department for a specific case.

The second time they met, Tim went by Priscilla's office to say a friendly hello. They were in the same subspecialty of litigation. Her office was a bit far from his, so he would occasionally pop by. Tim liked her; they had an instant rapport, as they practiced the same type of law. Tim had flirted with another lawyer in the firm, who had left, but that didn't go anywhere; however, he had a strong feeling for his new colleague and wasn't deterred.

To visit Priscilla, Tim used the excuse of dropping off a binder he had picked up at a conference. "Whenever he came by," said Priscilla, "I got giddy and avoided eye contact." Tim deferred. "She was quiet." Then he asked her to go to an outdoor Boston Pops concert at the first sign of the New England summer. Priscilla was attracted to Tim and thought he was nice, but "He was junior, and I never anticipated anything more."

Gradually, the couple got to know each other by going to social events at work over the course of several months. After two years they became engaged, but still kept their relationship secret. Priscilla told nobody at work, and Tim told only his best friend. Later, informed of the couple's engagement, Tim's boss, a partner, said, "I'm not stupid, I could tell you guys were involved." Similarly, a co-worker remarked to Priscilla: "It was the level of familiarity you had with each other at meetings that gave you away."

Secrecy meant one hopping out of the taxi and going into the building while the other paid and dawdled. It wasn't a game, explained Tim. Even if they had abided by the policy for office romance, *It wouldn't matter what the policy said if people were upset . . . I didn't want my boss to know because he goes off on people who demonstrate bad judgment. . . . Perhaps it was poor judgment to date within the firm, but the ends justified the means!*

During their first year of marriage, Priscilla became pregnant. They decided that she would be a stay-at-home mom, and that they would live in the town where they had bought a weekend summer place. Tim stayed in the city several nights a week. Their comments show what a magnificent team they are. "You miss work, you say that sometimes," said Tim to Priscilla. "I miss being at work with Tim," she said quietly, correcting him. "It's much lonelier for me at work now," said Tim. "My dream would be to have a practice with Priscilla. The work is a lot harder without her."

AN OFFICE ROMANCE THAT BEGAN AT A PICNIC

Janice, late thirties, is slim and fine-boned with long straight black hair, big, long-lashed dark eyes, and refined manners. She graduated from a small prestigious college in 1992 with a degree in history. "What's a girl to do with that? Go into retail, naturally!" She moved to the Philadelphia area, and began working in the management development program at Larkspur & Clothier's (L&C) flagship store in downtown Philadelphia. But that was a disappointment (and misnomer) because, according to Janice, in reality there was no management development: it was much more like slave labor, with very few weekends and holidays off. She did love her co-workers and the challenges of her position, but after two years decided to find a job that was "Monday to Friday, nine to five, like the rest of the world."

In 1993, Janice found a customer service position at EMQ, a telecommunications company also located in Philadelphia. Unlike L&C, EMQ was a relatively new company (only five years old) that had attracted a relatively young employee base. "Everyone was in their twenties, very good looking; and many people knew each other and had found jobs at EMQ via word of mouth. It was a very fun place to work."

The company was split into the operations groups, which were located in the center of Philadelphia, and the sales team, located in the outskirts of the city. Right from the start, Janice found her customer service colleagues to be a tight-knit group. They ate lunch together, chatted together, commiserated over miserable customers, hung out on the weekends, and just generally enjoyed one another.

In the spring, EMQ arranged softball games between operations and sales teams. Being in customer service, Janice dealt with the salespeople every day on the phone, but rarely saw them in person. The softball games were a popular social activity because the two departments were able to mix it up. After the games, there were usually parties; at these events, Janice explained:

> There was quite a lot of juicy gossip generated based on different people hooking up. It was easy to sort some people into stereotypical roles— office slut, office tease, office stud, and so forth. I think that one of the key elements that made these events so enjoyable was that we were all basically at the same point in our lives—young, single, no real responsibilities, living paycheck to paycheck, enjoying going out and having fun.

There were two corporate-sponsored social events, as well. In the fall, there was a company picnic. Most people either came by themselves or brought along friends, forming a happy and inviting group of people. Many relationships formed that way—friend of a friend of a friend. In December, there was the Christmas Party—an especially outstanding event because it was black tie. *Sometimes you didn't even recognize people right off the bat because they were so gussied up! The Christmas party was also an occasion for the company owners to recognize key employees with special awards, such as Employee of the Year, Team Player of the Year, and Manager of the Year.*

Seventeen years later and I still have many, many EMQ friends and connections. Over the years, my roommates have been friends from EMQ. Even when people left EMQ for another company, they were still part of the normal crowd. I guess in a way it sounds like a high school clique.

In the summer of 1993, Janice was with some college friends at a party in Princeton, New Jersey, at a popular eating, drinking, and dancing establishment. *Lo and behold, we ran into a whole pack of friends from EMQ. We were all dancing and having a great time together. I was very briefly introduced to a sales guy named Judd Peale. It definitely was not one of those moments where sparks fly, or you think to yourself "this is the one." In fact, it was a loud and crowded dance floor and he might not have even heard my name.*

The company picnic was held a month later. Janice brought her roommate Dana along. Dana had gone to college with Janice and was one of her best friends. Since neither had a steady beau, there was a general understanding between them that they would always attend each other's parties. They would give each other moral support and get to meet each other's co-workers, whom they had already heard so much about. At the picnic, Janice was again introduced to Judd. Her response was "Nice to meet you." Judd's response was "We've met before, at the party in Princeton last month." Janice thought Judd was good-looking and appealing; she figured she had really been in a fog that first time because she drew a complete blank on it. There was a little flirtatious chitchat before she and Dana moved on to chatting with another group of people. On the way home from the picnic, they discussed "every little detail of each person we spoke to, what they were wearing, and what they said" (including Judd).

A few weeks later, on "a giddy Friday afternoon," Janice was leaving a voicemail for one of the sales people that she supported. She happened to notice Jim's name on her list, too. One of the things he had joked about with her at the picnic was that he hated to get voicemails from her because it usually meant that one of his customers was canceling. Very impulsively, Janice dialed Judd's number and left him a voicemail, starting with how one of his largest customers had canceled. *I couldn't keep from giggling, so then I told him that a bunch of us were meeting for drinks at a place called Chasers on South Street on Saturday night, if he wanted to come, too. I wasn't sure if he'd even get the message and I really didn't give it another thought. . . .* Dana and Janice headed down to Chasers on Saturday night to meet up with the usual suspects. To Janice's surprise, Judd did show up, and brought along his good friend Mack. There was plenty of drinking, dancing, and laughing. At the end of the evening, Judd offered to drive Janice home. *Well, I had come with Dana and didn't even have my key on me. I was still giddy so I said okay. First we had to drive his friend Mack home. We went into Mack's house for a snack. While we were standing in the kitchen in front of the open refrigerator door, we had our first kiss. Mack walked in on that and just started laughing. He told us that Dana had told him in no uncertain terms that there was no way her friend was ever going to hook up with his friend.*

Judd and I kept our budding romance on the down low. Neither of us was interested in being fodder for the next gossip session. We didn't work directly together but our paths did cross. It was very exciting to have this special secret! However, I didn't want to get a reputation for being an office tramp, so if things didn't look like they were going to work out with Judd then I'd just as soon that no one else knew about it. The company Christmas party was held two months after we began dating. This was a dilemma: Did we go together, in which case everyone would know that we were dating, or did we go separately and continue the ruse by ignoring each other? In the end, we decided to go together. It did set tongues wagging, but in a good way. Everyone was so happy for us and thought that we were an adorable couple. A few years later, at the 1995 Christmas party, Judd was recognized as the Team Player of the Year and I received the Employee of the Year award. We were quite the EMQ power couple!

The sales team was awarded special trips as incentives. In the next five years, Judd and Janice went to Disney World, the Bahamas, Las Vegas, and Mexico. Factor in destination weddings for their other EMQ friends, and they did a lot of traveling together with their colleagues. *We became inseparable as a whole.*

In 1996, Judd very nervously took Janice to the restaurant where they had their first date and proposed to her. The following year, their families, friends, and EMQ colleagues joined them for a large, traditional wedding. A couple of years later, they had their first child, and then another. Said Janice:

> When I came back to work, I was splitting my time between working from home and the office. I didn't have an office anymore, just a cubicle. So I would go to Jim's office twice a day to pump breast milk.

In 2007, Janice was laid off when the company was acquired. When she found out the news, she said:

> I cried as if my best friend had just died. During those years, EMQ was such a constant in our lives. It was where I met my husband, which led to our two beautiful children. It was where many of my current friendships started. I didn't feel bitter, or regret a thing. I was just so happy

that I had the privilege of that experience. It's funny, I had gone to EMQ just to find a job where I could work Monday to Friday from nine to five, and what I found was a husband, two children, more friends than I can count, and a lifetime of memories.

LOVE THAT BEGAN IN A BAR

People meet and fall in love through work in a variety of venues—with outside contractors, at a convention, taking a break and chatting with an interesting person, flying to a meeting and sitting next to someone fascinating on the plane . . . all these situations are work related. In this book, we focus on the traditional company/office workplace and relationships that spring up between co-workers. But as people also fall in love with in every business, from "both sides of the counter," and as the workplace can be virtually anything that people are doing, the broader perspective is also meaningful. Therefore, we include a sample romance from a broader definition of the word "workplace" . . . retail sales to customers, librarians who deal with the public, waitresses and patrons, or health provider and patient.

Bettina sat in her corner office in one of the top publishing companies in the world. She came from a suburban town in a Southern state and dreamed of life in Manhattan. Her parents and sisters were proud of her and she was moving up the corporate ladder, but this wasn't the New York she had dreamed of; it was, well, just another desk job. She was dating an actor, and that did spice things up, but he was head over heels in love with himself. So she began to take acting classes, and, at 34, announced to her parents she was going to become an actress.

"At 34?," her mother screamed. "If your sister wanted to do this, fine, she's 24, but you, Tina, are too old!"

That was the last Bettina and her parents communicated for some time. Meanwhile, she took acting classes, got a role in an off-Broadway production as an ingénue, and, pro forma, earned her keep as a waitress, first at a chic bistro that hired beautiful dancers. However, because she sometimes practiced lines in her head and forgot orders, she went to work in a trendy bar near the NYU medical center.

A young intern who was too busy to have a girlfriend used to come in and talk with her. Mostly Bettina knew to cut short the customers' palaver, but she and Shawn, the intern, quickly became buddies. He would come and eat his quick supper at the bar, and especially liked to hear her stories of acting class, auditions, and such. He was from southern California, and except for Bettina's hilarious stories, was not tuning in much to the Big Apple.

Then Shawn got a residency in San Diego. Bettina missed him but was philosophical—he was a patron of where she worked, basically, and they had not seen each other outside it. But Shawn suddenly missed Bettina acutely. No one else could make him laugh like she could, and few had her energy and love of life. He began to phone her. When she told him she had mononucleosis, that was his cue to fly back from San Diego, take care of her, and as she said, "like a hero in a romance novel," propose on bended knee.

A year later and boom, boom, they have a child and Bettina has made another nonconventional career move to designing and marketing original, high-quality baseball hats—with Shawn's involvement and support. "It all happened so quickly I didn't know what hit me," said Bettina. "For years I languished in my job, doing the right thing, and was pretty cynical about the men I dated. Then I became a bartender and met a truly decent, brilliant man who respected me for myself, not a label." Bettina thinks that working in a service job was an important element to the romance. *Romances need hurdles, and ours was overcoming a stereotype on both sides. He reminded me of the handsome doctors on daytime TV and he says that I had the attitude and look of Claire Danes in* Me and Orson Welles, *his fantasy movie about New York. But I'm intellectual and crack jokes, and he's quirky and far from omniscient, so the getting-to-know you phase lasted a long time.*

In a bar, where loose manners and hitting on the girl bartender are a tradition, how did Bettina keep the interpersonal, male-female relations pleasant? What can she recommend based on her experience on how to behave/interact with male clients at work—to not cross over the line to being personal, yet show "interest" or attraction when there is a special person who comes into your workplace and has "date potential"?

I was very prim and proper at the bar; in fact, at the beginning, I was naive. Shawn was only my third boyfriend, and I was friendly to everybody when I began the job. We'd talk and the men would say they would love to continue the conversation and ask for my phone number and I would give it, thinking it was strictly platonic. Then I got better at drawing the line. I'd have a short conversation and be a good listener but I learned the trick of not letting them know anything personal about me.

The owner encouraged us to drink to be in a good mood. I didn't because I had strict notions about both relationships and work. So when Shawn asked me out—it was my first shift and he'd just moved to New York to do his residency, I said no . . . *"It's not proper, thank you—you're a customer." But he lived around the corner and came in often. When I conversed with him he thought I was being nice and I thought I was flirting. Then after a few months, he said, 'I'd like to ask you out but you will think I'm hitting on you so forget I asked. . . . I was going to say yes this time but he left without hearing me!*

Don't expect to have a romance of consequence with someone you serve a drink or a meal to at a public establishment. This is why it took several years, and my moving away, for Shawn and me to come together—the locale and the situation definitely held things back. I didn't want to be regarded as an attractive woman to hang out with, like a stripper, which is the attitude of male clients to women who are in jobs like mine. After all, at this bar I was hired because the owner liked an exotic-looking women. But if you become friends to a certain level, where you count on each other and feel affection, that's the basis for love no matter where you work.

By patience and having sterling character, untangled the client of a customer hitting on an attractive worker in the service industry and braided a beautiful love.

IN LOVE IN D.C.

Seeing poor job prospects in academics, Aaron left the divinity program at Yale for business school in the South. When he got a job as a "consultant, government practice" in D.C., worked like the devil to make the switch. A friend from business school worked on the fifth floor, and when he walked down one day to chat with her, there was another woman at a desk whom Aaron couldn't help but notice:

> The suit she was wearing was canary yellow. She wore a silk scarf, large gold bangles, and black pumps. I gaped and she typed. She had beautiful hands with long, tapering fingers, lovely features on the sensual side, and a husky voice that I overheard on the phone.

Nothing happened at this juncture except that their eyes met. Looking back, Aaron said that he had a visceral response that his thoughts couldn't interpret. *I didn't know her, but I stayed focused on her, even with all the other available women in the office, and in other places I went. It all sounds vague, but that's how things begin sometimes. I had a sturdy build, I dressed well, and I was okay looking, but I never had women falling all over me. This relationship would require time and patience—I knew that. The singular difference is that I had an image of her in my head that didn't go away.*

I went away again for a few weeks on an assignment, and then returned to the city. I went to see my friend down the hall again, this time on a different pretext. I began to ask her questions: "Do you know her? Is she dating anyone? What do you think?" At this point I got the look that all women give to men ... "Why don't you ask her (stupid)?"

Aaron asked Suzanne out for a drink, and she said "yes." They saw each other occasionally over the next few weeks. She already had a social life, since she had grown up in the area. All the same, she was available to go out to dinner when Aaron asked.

During one of those times, they were seen by someone in the office, and one of the other consultants warned Aaron, "No dating in the office." Aaron ignored this, "as if I'd never heard it, but I did mention it to Suzanne." From then on, they stopped holding hands a block before they came to the office, and left at different times to go to the same place. *Professional decorum always prevailed inside of the office. The romance stayed a secret between a few friends and us. We got to know each other, to find out about personal history, and family, and foibles.* They cooked at each other's apartments, went to the steeplechases in Virginia, on an overnight trip to an antebellum mansion, met each other's families, and signed "love" on daily letters they wrote when Aaron was on a long business trip in Portland, Oregon.

A year passed. Aaron was thinking about a ring. Then, when he returned from the trip, he heard the news he had been expecting. The workload had decreased. People were being let go as soon as their last project was finished. He and Suzanne were both let go (within a year the partnership dissolved) and were jobless. *Any thought of marriage was on hold while we both went through the ordeal of looking for a job in a metropolitan area with tens of thousands of highly educated people.*

This put stress on the relationship. Since it could not go forward, Aaron explained, it threatened to stall from the stress and uncertainty: *I felt like I couldn't provide the proper security and financial support to carry a marriage.*

Suzanne, predictably, being more focused on a career area (personnel management) than Aaron, found a job first, about five months later. On her first day driving into work, she got into a bad automobile accident and fractured bones in her right foot. Now it was Aaron who put the sock on her cast every morning as she left for work and massaged her swollen foot every evening. He found a job a month later. Once they were both employed again, they moved forward with their wedding plans. Then Suzanne was dubbed by a boss at the old firm for a much higher-level job, and as she was recruiting for positions, met people who did executive placement. This led to a permanent position for Aaron. Despite many setbacks they were on track. *We decided to take the final step and complete the picture of our lives as we imagined it would be. We put our town house on the market, bought a home with a cherry tree in the front yard, and Suzanne got pregnant.* Now they decided they could live on Aaron's salary alone.

The story of Aaron and Suzanne is very typical of young professionals who meet at work. In a past generation, the female would have been the secretary; now the woman had a job opportunity equal to the man's. They chose to return to the classic model of a marriage, where the woman stays home with the children. However, their expectation consisted of her possibly going back to work and his possibly going back to academics, i.e., the model looked the same on the outside but was shot with a contemporary attitude about both career and role flexibility.

ACADEMIC AFFAIR

After being in the Air Force, Jose went back to school and earned a Ph.D. in social work. He was an assistant professor at a university in California, divorced with no children, when he met Laura (who was on the nursing faculty). She was in an unhappy marriage. Her husband was a physician: he was never available and did not want children. She wanted a companion, and time was running out on her biological clock.

It was love at first sight, said Jose when he met her on a curriculum committee to which they had both been assigned. Laura had not thought of ending her marriage, and her enjoyment when interacting with Jose before and after the curriculum meeting (which did not meet often enough for her) took her by surprise.

Jose invited Laura for lunch—she went, and sparks flew. Fast forward: Laura divorced her husband, Jose and Laura married, and the couple both got jobs at a university in Texas, closer to Laura's parents. They now have two sons and a private practice in divorce mediation (in addition to their university positions).

PEOPLE OF THE THEATER

Valerie Vigoda and Brendan Milburn are two of the three stars of the production company Groove Lily, which has created and performed numerous original musicals that have toured the country in the last 10 years, including Broadway. They were interviewed from the "Toy

Story" rehearsal hall in Anaheim, California, where they were switching off each day so one of them could take care of their son. *We are accustomed to being together in situations like this so it is quite usual,* said Valerie.

Brendan related the story of how they met and fell in love, and how they work together as a couple. *I wanted it to be romance from the get-go—I saw Val play and sing at a club called "Tramps" in New York City in 1994—and I fell hard for her that night. I bought her CD, met her at a party afterward, and wormed my way into a conversation with her by finding and playing Journey's "Lovin', Touchin', Squeezin'" on the tape player. I was certain that she was the kind of person who would dig me if I sang along with the harmonies at the end. It was totally corny, but I was right. It worked. Her interest was piqued.*

We started writing songs together before we started dating—but only barely. She was convinced I was gay, and I had been told by a mutual friend that she had vowed never to date another younger man, and especially not a younger musician. Plus, I was playing happy-hour piano in a gay bar on Christopher Street, studying writing musical theater, and I'm from San Francisco—so Val was convinced that I was her new gay friend Brendan.

She'd finally worked up the courage to tell me, "I know you're gay, but I just have to tell you that I find you really attractive and I don't want to ruin our budding friendship." I interrupted and told her, "I know you're not interested in dating younger men, or musicians, but . . ." And then we stayed up all night and watched the sun come up on the roof of her apartment building, and drank tea, and had our first kiss. It was awesome. We've been playing music and writing songs together since about a week or two after we've met, and that was over 15 years ago.

Being a couple is at dead center of their creations. According to Brendan:

> It can be great, and it can be terrible. When you're married to the person you work with creatively, it feels like the creative highs are multiplied exponentially—a big break, a great song, a wonderful new idea, a success—these things become so much more wonderful and joyous as a result of being able to share them together.
>
> Sadly, this means that the crappy moments are made more so by having both members of the partnership experience them simultaneously. I know there have been times when each of us has wished we'd married some nice doctor whose life, with its many highs and lows, wasn't in perfect sync with ours.
>
> In addition, it's not just emotional highs and lows that are magnified—all the financial woes are made much worse because we both have all of our eggs in the same baskets. It can be very tough.

For a collaboration to be a working two-way street, you need to have trust, faith, and respect for the other person, even when your spouse is telling you that you just had the worst idea in the world, and it needs to be thrown away. A large part of what we do is to tell each other to go back and do better, and our creative work is so much better as a result of this.

TWO WORLD-CLASS ASTROPHYSICISTS

When I heard about Ned and Ellen, I [Jane] asked them to join me for breakfast. I drove up to Boston in a snowstorm to interview them, feeling that this was the poster couple of our book for several reasons. They are both equally strong, have amazing backgrounds, had varied experiences before marriage, they love their work, and they would not have come together in, say, college or high school, although they are beautifully matched. They started the relationship as friends, and they are starry-eyed in love. In person, Ned and Ellen struck me with their high intelligence, humility, and good humor.

The star imagery comes to mind because Ned and Ellen are astrophysicists who met in their research institute. Ned had done a lot of trekking and wandering the world before he applied his astrophysics Ph.D. to a real job. Ellen came to the institute by way of a responsible, high-tech position in the military.

Ned and his officemate, Tom, who had recently married, were sitting in their office one day when a program manager brought Ellen by. It was her first day. A lot of the researchers worked with their doors open unless they were in certain purlieus; however, recently Tom and Ned had agreed to keep their door closed because, as Tom observed, Ned was so popular that everybody was always stopping by to say hello.

Ellen was a breath of fresh air—radiant, with a big smile on her face, Ned recalled. She had a friendly countenance, and she was pretty in a distinctive way, with honey-colored skin, and symmetrical, delicate features in a rounded face. That not many women worked in their program meant that when they saw an attractive woman, the guys checked her out. Ned and Tom gave each other a look when Ellen left, but Ned said, "Did you see the ring?"

Ned, Tom and Ellen started working together on a project. They spent several weeks on data collection campaigns still early in their friendship (and it was that experience that helped Ned and Ellen get to know each other). Then Tom, who usually traveled on missions to an observatory with Ned, stopped traveling on such campaigns because of young fatherhood—leaving Ellen and Ned to coordinate and execute them as a pair. Now Ned and Ellen were not only working at the observatory, but were out doing a field experiment in the desert—virtually looking at the starry sky together at night.

Ellen had been an Army officer, and was accustomed to getting along in a mostly male work environment. Her parents were Hispanic: her father was an Army pastor who grew up in Texas, and her mother was a social worker who had immigrated from Hong Kong. Their first languages were Spanish and Chinese, but Ellen had been raised in their common language, English, to be a "very American patriot." Ellen had strong religious values, as well. Ned was from Ohio. His dad was an engineer, and his mom a homemaker. He had the look of a blond jock but possesses an awesome brain for math and science, and a love of the stars. They discovered that while their backgrounds were disparate, there were also commonalities: Ellen was the oldest of four daughters and Ned was the oldest of four sons, and they were both from loving, close, education-oriented families. Currently, both were in relationships. Ellen was engaged to a software engineer who had recently been hired to work at the institute. Ned had an unsatisfying, long-distance relationship that had gone on without resolution for three years. Ellen normally dated people she knew very well through work. Her fiancé was the exception. At 34, she was ready to settle down, Her fiancé had appeared on the scene, was affable, worked in a field contiguous to hers, and was open to religious faith, which also impressed her. *I fell in love with that portion of this guy in particular*, she said. When they got engaged, they bought a large house together. Her younger sister and niece moved in with them for a year while her sister was looking for work.

Said Ned, *We were technical collaborators, doing monkey work at the observatory and numbers work in the institute. We found we worked well together—that evolved along with our friendship. It's hard to imagine Ellen as a tough Army woman, because she's feminine and vulnerable. I was blown away. She is the ultra mix.* Ellen commented: *I put on a uniform when I go to the institute just as I did in the Army. I was struck by Ned's emotional intelligence and how observant he is.*

When Ned's relationship went sour, he went to his pal Ellen for support. He would take time out of the working day to see Ellen. Meanwhile, Tom, who loved systems, influenced Ned to chart how many days before he called his ex: *I graphed everything. My recovery was a huge part of my day.* Ellen said: *He puts his all into a relationship. That impressed me.* Ned would sit down and say if he was having a tough day. Ellen never got the vibe that he was interested in her, beyond a source of empathy and friendship.

Despite the nights under the starry sky, it was platonic between Ned and Ellen. In fact, Ellen helped Ned find other people to date. She advised him to delete his picture from an online dating site (after which he averred that he had more success). Tom had advised Ned to come to Internet dates with back-up talking points, and Ned sometimes reviewed with Ellen the topics he could talk about in a conversational lull.

In the process of confiding in each other, they both discovered that they were loyal to a fault. Neither of them ever considered leaving their partner for each other. Once Tom said, "Listen, dude, you and Ellen need to be together," but Ned says he didn't really hear it. *I didn't even emotionally entertain the idea. She'd give me pointers for whomever I was dating that month.* She and her fiancé were going through the stress of having her sister and children in their household, and Ellen talked to Ned about that.

Then Ellen's fiancé went from throwing temper tantrums to attacking her. The second time, she ended up with a broken lip. She knew it was over between them, but with their shared real estate, it was going to take a while to get free. When she went into work the day after he injured her, Ellen went to Ned. She recalled, *I was in a haze at work and figured that if I didn't tell someone it would not be a reality.* When Ned saw that Ellen wasn't wearing her ring, he knew that she was leaving the relationship, irreversibly. *I tempered my reaction, but even though she is such a loyal person, I believed she would not give her fiancé another chance.* Ned said to call him if there was more trouble. Ellen felt, along with being traumatized by her fiancé's behavior, that she could now break the engagement. *When my sister said to be happy that he hadn't hit me with a two-by-four for me to call it quits, that was eye-opening.*

Meanwhile, Ned reproved himself for selfishly thinking that Ellen might be "single in six months." He broke up with his casual girlfriend, feeling bad about that because there was no reason, except that he would never forgive himself if he didn't become available for Ellen. He kept his plan/designs secret except for telling one brother, to whom he said, 'I'm going to wait it out. This is the kind of girl I dreamed of to be my wife.'

The coming together took time. They both had a free day a couple of weeks after Ellen broke off her engagement. She decided to go to work, as her fiancé was still living in the house. She told Ned that she had all kinds of work to do, and, lo and behold, Ned came in as well. The institute was virtually empty. *I had to tell her how I felt. I was as nervous as I've ever been, just tragic, but I knew I had to do it. I said, "Hey, let's grab lunch." The cafeteria was closed, so it was an opportunity to be with her away from the institute and away from work. Basically, I sat in my office for three hours waiting until lunch, when she told me about the changes in her life. There was no opportune moment to make my statement. Then we were back in the building. I dumbly followed her into her office and sat in her chair. I'd had my speech planned during lunch, and if I didn't say it then, then when? So, at last, as I was going out the door, I said, "I just want you to know, when you are ready to date, I want to be the first in line." And Ellen stared at me, as though a tidal wave had hit her.*

Ellen said: *We both had real backburner stuff. And I'm not his type. He was one of those guys who dated women who were cute, blonde, about 5'6", sleek, and slender.*

Ellen was floored. Ned was happy he had said something, and went back and sat again in his office for two hours, practically immobilized. Then she came by, with a big smile and a blush on her face, and their relationship transmuted from friendship to romance with one extended look of love. *It was goofy,* Ned chuckled. Ned told Ellen he would wait for her, and didn't press her to change her state of mind (which was in a breakup phase).

If they had been in another context, now that they were both free to give their hearts, they would have sailed into a dating spree. But this was a workplace they loved, and they were even on the same team. Plus, Ellen was still feeling fragile after the nightmarish conclusion to her engagement with another man. Two weeks later, they went out on a dinner date, but, according to Ellen, *We were both looking over our shoulders the whole time.* But now Ned was bursting with love. He said to his brother, *This is the type of girl who has all the qualities, who meets my minimum requirements. I have felt an incremental growth of love for her.* Laughing at Ned's "nerdy" declaration of his affection, his brother said, "I know you'll marry her."

Ellen is serious and not impetuous. Like Ned, her devotion to ethics is her North Star. She was truly astonished by Ned's romantic interest, yet she had, dispassionately, already held him in high esteem, and thought the woman who ended up with him would be fortunate indeed. "Ned is independent and caring. I wanted kids, and he had that appealing quality that appeals to me of being a kid himself—in a good way."

Working in the same group at the institute, Ellen and Ned proceeded with caution. *We didn't know if it was cool for us to be a couple,* said Ellen. Still, they were hiding the romance. "We were beginning to see each other. One day we were at a mall and Ned, who has incredible face recognition, saw our group leader at the other end of Macy's, coming in with his children. Without a moment's reflection I dodged to one side and hid behind a rack of clothes. I hid as he came down the aisle. I thought I'd be able to handle it, but I couldn't!"

Then Ned had a discussion with the group leader. The leader closed the door of the office and asked, "So, what's going on?" Ned has a way of lighting up, and said something like, "What do you need to know?" The group leader nodded and said, "I got all I need to know—and it's fine." Commented Ned: *It reminded me of when my dad came and said, "You know all about the birds and the bees, right?"*

When it's said that two scientists work on the same team, it means that they work closely. For instance, on occasion Ellen and Ned do "pair programming," where they program at one work station. One types in code and one reviews it line by line. They switch roles every half hour or so (the pair-programming method is used to create more elegant designs, and it allows knowledge to pass between the two programmers).

When they began to work together as a romantic couple, there were subtle changes. When Ned told Ellen to make sure that she did something in a certain way, she was now a bit on the alert that he wasn't commanding her. They agree that they had (as Ned put it) "a couple of speed bumps" on a project, where they threw up their hands and brought their personal emotions in when they were "in work mode." He said, *The emotional part of our relationship became part of our work life. There didn't seem to be a way around that and at some point the fusion just got much better. We had challenges at first, but also found a new forum in which to discuss things. Now even though we brought emotions into our science, we could close the door and have a personal discussion at work that helped on the work and relationship fronts. One of us could say, "I was hurt that you thought it wouldn't work." We had a new plane on which to develop a work relationship because we weren't afraid of being personal or emotional.*

Ellen was the more hesitant to critique and express feelings about their work, at work, but Ned said if they left a "spot on the lens" they would both be tense. *I'd say, "Let's take 20 minutes now to talk about it," and Ellen adapted, and added an approach of "because we don't carry any negativity home with us."* On several instances over the last two years, their door was closed and they were at their workstations having it out professionally and emotionally. Consequently, they have seen their personal dynamics only improve.

They attest that they help each other out while preparing for technical presentations, providing feedback on the content and script. Said Ned, *It's easier to do that with a mate than with a colleague sometimes, because you can be more honest and direct. However, it's a chicken-and-egg scenario, in that while you're honest and direct, you have to keep a keener eye on the sensitivity of the other.*

Despite how busy one of them may be at any given time, they make time for each other, whether it's technical or personal. Driving home from work in the car together is their preferred time to debrief on the workday, and typically, *When we arrive home we're all done with that, and are ready to enjoy our social life together.*

Over three years of working together, falling in love, and marrying, Ned and Ellen have proved to each other and to others that they are a force as a working couple. The institute has sent them on missions to solve problems at observatories together, and their reputations in their field have risen in tandem. When I interviewed them, they were just starting to work on different projects with different people more often, so they saw less direct collaboration happening in the near future. *This will probably be a good thing*, said Ned. *Our work relationship may morph into a hello-wanna-grab-a-coffee or let's-do-lunch kind of thing, with the ability to escape with each other when we need it. That's something we try not to take for granted, as we know most of the other astronomers don't get that kind of opportunity.* Added Ellen, *But we also try not to flaunt it, of course!*

That they are one of several couples at the institute helps; according to Ellen, others have "paved the way." But a disadvantage that Ellen expressed was that the institute does tend to be all-consuming. It has a fitness center, Ned bowls in an institute league, and they have beach parties and ski trips with colleagues. Most of the scientists are young and from elsewhere in the country and their whole social circle is made up of other scientists and engineers at the institute. *We speak about it but don't stress about it*, said Ellen. *We look what's happening in our area on the weekend and do a lot of random, fun events. When we have kids, we would like to be around Ned's family or mine. He and his brothers dream of having a engineering business, but it would be hard to give up work that is as exhilarating as ours.*

DATING MY MANAGER TURNED OUT TO BE A DISASTER

This story comes from a technical consultant for *Fortune* 500 companies, who is female, and in her late 40s.

Yes, I dated someone whom I met at work. It took about 10 months before we had a relationship because I was dating someone else. But I was very attracted to him from the moment I saw him. Once we got together, the relationship went on for two years. It ended because he had a relationship with a much younger woman while we were engaged—it was easier for him to have an affair and create a rift than to just be honest and break off the engagement. Such an immature coward. So while I was willing at first to work through the issues and get married, I realized it was never going to work. In retrospect, it was a big mistake. I wasted two years of my life on someone who really didn't know what he wanted and did not know what commitment was. Yes, it changed the way I felt about my job, which I really enjoyed and through which I had earned a lot of credibility and respect. During the relationship, we realized that we could not have a manager/employee work relationship, so he moved into another department. After we broke up, I just wanted to get away.

I was very much infatuated and wanted to marry him. We were both single, he was divorced. At first we kept the relationship secret. And when he changed departments, we dated openly, even though by then I suspect most people in our office knew what was going on.

I did not want others to know about it at all.

Yes, I also dated a client of sorts after this relationship. At first I refused to go out with him because he was a client and it would be unprofessional. However, he was extremely persistent. He said he was really just a consultant for the client, so he wasn't really a customer. And it was flattering. So, we dated for several months.

Believe me, I always felt that dating someone from your workplace was a big mistake. So it's pretty ironic that I ended up obsessively in love with my manager, and that the whole thing ended up being a disaster.

The only person I've ever worked with and had a crush on was this man. And I acted on it. It escalated very quickly; we had sex on the first night that we got together.

Had the affair been open, I think it would've been less exciting because there is always something more romantic or stimulating when the relationship is illicit.

I felt extremely not guilty, but I was doing something that people could raise as an issue if they found out and wanted to be difficult. And probably most people knew, it was not a big office. But as a result, when I had evidence of another colleague's gross incompetence/dishonesty, I felt at a disadvantage. I could not call this person out on it, because the response might have been "What right do you have? You're having an affair with your manager?" Then the whole affair would be out, and my perfect image tarnished. It is stupid now, in retrospect, to have worried, but when you're very young and new to the work place, you want to do everything right, show good judgment. And having a relationship with your manager is very, very bad judgment.

So I think that was also why I was determined to marry him, to show everyone that it wasn't just a fling, that it was a serious relationship where our feelings transcended the conventions of work. Marriage would justify my stepping outside the rules. Personally, I was just obsessively unhealthily in love.

When I went to work in a different office, there were a high number of single young professionals under the age of 30. As a result, there were many relationships and office dramas. There was no official policy prohibiting office romance, I suppose, because all the young people were peers. There wasn't much opportunity for one person to take advantage of another, or for one person to influence someone else's professional success.

The stories in this chapter reveal the range of experiences in the workplace: from those who met and married to those who ended up leaving a firm over a failed love affair. In general, the risks of an office affair are minimal, and the outcome is usually deliriously positive. The exception is when a boss and subordinate have an affair. Where there is considerable risk, the loser will be the subordinate.

15

Being in Business/Working Together

Partnership, not dependence, is the real romance in marriage.
                                                    Muriel Fox Aronson

Office lovers who become spouses are in for some changes. Whether both spouses stay on a career path with the same company, one spouse quits while the other remains with the company, or both spouses quit and go into business together, their marriage is a catalyst for fresh thinking and altered lives. We begin this chapter with a review of how money and marriage interface.

MONEY AND MARRIAGE

Money is a central issue in marriage because of its association with power, control, and dominance. Generally, the more money a spouse makes, the more power he or she has in the relationship. Men make considerably more money than do women. The average annual income of a man with some college who is working full-time is $48,993, compared with $36,836 for a woman with the same education, also working fulltime, year-round.[1] Yet, two researchers found that although two-thirds of the husbands (in a national sample) in dual-income marriages said that they made more money than do their wives, women were still more likely to make the decisions in more areas (42% versus 30%).[2]

When the wife has an income, her sway in the relationship increases. Let's consider the frequent scenario when a wife (who had stayed home with the kids) goes back to work. Before her first paycheck, her husband's fishing boat was parked in the protected carport of the couple's home. With her new job, and increased power in the relationship, she began to park her car in the carport, and her husband parked his fishing boat underneath the pine trees to the side of the house.

Money also provides an employed woman with the wherewithal to be independent and not to be forced to marry a man to pay her bills. Money also allows an employed woman to leave an unhappy marriage. Indeed, the higher a wife's income, the more likely she is to leave an unhappy relationship.[3]

To some individuals, money reflects love. While admiring her friend's twenty-fifth anniversary ring, a woman, said, "What a big diamond! He must really love you." The implication behind the statement reflects the cultural assumption that a large, expensive diamond equals a lot of sacrifice and love.

WHEN THERE ARE TWO CAREERS IN ONE MARRIAGE

A dual-career marriage is defined as one in which both spouses pursue careers. A career is distinct from a job, in that the former usually involves advanced education or training, full-time commitment, working nights or weekends "off the clock," and a willingness to relocate. Dual-career couples operate without a "wife"—a person who stays home to manage the household and care for children and/or dependents.

When a couple has traditional gender role attitudes, or the couple simply takes a hard look at their respective salaries or earning potentials, the husband's career is likely to take precedence. This situation often results in the wife's willingness to relocate and to disrupt her career for the advancement of her husband's career. In a study of 36 professional women, the husband's career took precedence in 22 percent of their marriages.[4]

The primary reasons for this arrangement were that the husband's higher salary (it was easier for the couple to go where the husband could earn the highest income since the wife could find a job wherever he went), and ego needs (the husband wished to have the dominant career). This arrangement is sometimes at the expense of the wife's career. A common example is the wife who moves wherever her military husband is assigned, thus disrupting her career (often over and over).

Another traditional scenario is when the wife gets pregnant, stops working, and stays home to rear the children. The problem with two careers in one marriage is that there is no "wife" to provide a backup for the respective workers. Shopping, preparing meals, and taking care of the house all take time, which two career-driven individuals have little time for.

Other couples agree that it is the wife's career that will take precedence (HER/his). Still others regard their careers equally (HIS/HER), or both spouses share a career, or work together in a business.

WORK AND LIFE: CREATING AN EQUAL PARTNERSHIP

Some couples operate a small business together. Indeed, family-owned businesses make up 80 to 90 percent of companies in the U.S. and employ almost half of the workforce; couple-owned businesses account for the majority of new businesses.[5] One researcher [6] examined entrepreneurial couples, coined the term "co-preneurs," and identified nine traits that couples who managed the interface between a business and personal relationship share: marriage and children come first; they have spousal respect for each other; there is open/effective communication; the partners' talents complement each other; the partners are supportive of each other; spouses have strong family ties; spouses compete with the outside world, not with each other; spouses like to laugh; and the spouses keep their egos in check.

One example is a couple that has a furniture business together on a quaint main street in New England. Each helps the other, doing what the *Book of Common Prayer 1662* calls "works of supererogation" for each other. The husband and wife build four-poster beds together with each installing wood bolts to the exact, down-to-the millimeter tightness. This is their livelihood, but they also enjoy seeing one of their pieces of furniture find a home.

The wife we interviewed spoke of participating in a crafts fair and their enjoyment in spending the weekend together, even though it was not much different than their day-to-day furnituremaking enterprise and management of the store. Couples who leave the grind of working for someone else and pursue an enterprise together delight in their independence and shared venture.

Jane (first author) once persuaded her fiancé to build a marionette theater and a dozen stringed marionettes. She and her partner created puppets at night, like Geppetto, and performed in the days and evenings. They also joined a traveling theater, selling their hand puppets in a shop. Alas, they returned to day jobs, but enjoyed that unique time of having their own business venture.

The concept of merging work and relationships dates back to the thirteenth century, to the age of troubadours in France. At that time, the troubadour Chretien de Troyes wrote *Erec et Enide*, in which when the typical knight saw and fought for a lovely damsel, which turned out to be only the beginning of their relationship. Both the knight and the damsel had to problem solve and wield weapons to get out of the forest and back to the court so they could marry. And that only provided them with the rudimentary tools of marriage—step one in this depiction of de Troyes' ideal partnership.

What happens next is that Enide hears court gossip that Erec has been sloughing off since he married her. As the narrative goes, "He had no desire to joust. His only wish was to lie beside his wife, whom he made his sweetheart and his mistress. Embracing her and kissing her occupied all his attention, and he longed for no other pleasure."[7] So Enide confronts her young husband about his lack of desire for any activity outside of her, and his retort is essentially, "What, you don't appreciate my performance in bed?" To raise their identity as a couple from fatuous to brilliant, they decide to work together—literally. Now Erec takes Enide out with him on travels fraught with hostile and unpredictable enemies. By the end of their adventures, Erec has proven himself as more than just good in bed, and Enide has proven that she is just as capable of facing life's trials as Erec. Erec says to his bride: "My sweet sister, I have tested you in all ways. Now you have nothing more to fear, for now I love you more than ever. And I am again sure and certain of your perfect love for me."[8]

The practice of meeting your mate in the workplace or choosing to work as husband and wife in a business together has been present in preindustrial crafts for thousands of years. For example, regarding the highly developed weaving of Central and Western Asia, scholar John Wertime said that "in the totality of rug production, men and women usually did different things on a village and nomadic pastoralist level, where carpet weaving was almost exclusively a female pursuit. Men often sheared the sheep while women spun it, etc. In villages, men also did hand spinning. Spinning on machines was a male task in cities. There were male weavers of cloth in the villages and cities, usually in workshops, not in homes, where women wove. Workshop weaving was often a male pursuit, but not exclusively so, as males and females have also sat side by side in a collaborative effort."[9]

In the fifties and sixties in the United States, corporations focused as much on the wife as the husband in selecting their executives.

Corporations took steps to insure that their executives had "suitable" wives, including interviews in their homes or evaluating the sociability of wives at corporate parties. Some corporations provided seminars for the wives on how to be a good corporate helpmate. William Whyte, *Fortune* magazine editor stated in his book, *The Organization Man,* that "most wives agreed with the corporation: they too felt that the good wife is the wife who adjusts graciously to the system, curbs open intellectualism or the desire to be alone."[10] Today, women (and men) view themselves as equals in developing joint business ventures or professional services.

Some Hollywood couples reflect the union of career and marriage. Paul Newman and Joanne Woodward co-starred together and directed each other. (Woodward directed Newman in productions right up to the end of his life.) The couples who have worked together in the theater give us hints at what being married to your work partner really requires—what you have to give to it and what it gives back.

THE POWER SHIFT

When office lovers become a married couple, a third entity is formed: the relationship. There's the husband, the wife, and the couple. Relationship counselor Leigh Cousins commented: "The relationship is born in the overlap of the two people, but it definitely takes on a life of its own."[11] Management must now consider what the spouse will do if one member of the dyad gets a raise or a transfer. Co-workers now relate to each of them as part of a couple. If one is invited to an event, the other is included, or an explanation is due.

REAL-LIFE COUPLES WHO COMBINE WORK AND LOVE

The more that two people are established in their careers as mature adults, the less likely that one's interests get lost or overpowered by the other. Barbara Damrosch met and consulted with Eliot Coleman as one well-known authority on gardening to another. She traveled from Connecticut to see him at his Maine estate and was enthralled by his investigative, low-key approach to his unique northern crops. Then they kissed, and she had barely put down her straw bonnet before they married. Said Damrosch, "His garden is now 'our' garden, though I am only vice president when it comes to the vegetables (he is vice president of flowers).[12] Through their books on gardening, their readers can feel the spirit of their lives. As Thoreau said, "Good for the body is the work of the body, good for the soul the work of the soul, and good for either the work of the other."[13]

Couples who meet at the office, may find it plausible to leave the office together to chart their own path. *The Opt-Out Revolution*, by management expert Lisa A. Maniero, notes that men and women often follow a more relational rather than business model. *The tendency is to shift their neat upward and onward career pattern to rearrange their roles and relationship outside the corporate radar. Most couples who meet at the workplace are not going to continue in parallel lines; what they experience from the corporation is "here's the standard contract, like it or lump it." What they end up doing is leaving the firm, the rigid rules, and contracts.*[14]

Another scenario is that individuals meet and already have careers going. Once they marry, things change. Gabe and Natalie met and married. Her teaching career took a back seat (she quit) to raising their child. Gabe's business was doing well and he needed help. Natalie had always appreciated Gabe's work and had contributed in various ways, including grant-writing, and now she offered to take on the business management side for Gabe. Gabe, when interviewed, spoke of their dual partnership in work and marriage.

Natalie has been a much valued partner. Our field is on a fast track of R&D and the nature of how water is regulated. From my point of view, her work with me, and her teaching and planning skills have made it possible for me to excel in my learning. To have an arrangement like ours, it helps to be a certain type of person—to have personality traits such as being able to listen, open to new ideas, not argumentative, and able to focus. You also should like what you do.

Another example is a couple who work at the same university. An admissions director at a prestigious New England prep school said:

> My husband works in a different office at the same school, but because it's such a small environment (under 300 students total), I still feel we work in the same workplace. We are both administrators and coaches (not to mention that he is also a dorm parent!), so our day rarely ends at 5 or 6 p.m., like most office jobs do. We try to catch up for 20 minutes during lunch or dinner. While this might sound like a disadvantage, it's actually a nice perk. We live and work on the same campus, so we always know that the other person is nearby if we need anything. And even if we don't have time to talk for an extended period during the day, I will usually see him once or twice!
>
> Our hard work results in a better life for the other person. I mean that when I'm doing my best professionally (and for the school), my

husband directly benefits. The same is true in his position as dean of students. When he is doing well, I directly benefit. There is no one I trust more than my husband to put everything into what he does and help the greater good in our small school community.

The downside is that since we are both very passionate about our jobs and the school where we live and work, we will often carry our work stories home. We're each other's sounding board and we typically will talk about work for at least part of the evening. He knows when I've had a difficult day, and I know when he prefers to get off-campus to get away from it all. Only being married four years, we know this about each other. For some couples, this could take a lifetime, but because we work and live together, we read each other very well.

FERTILE MINDS

Married couple Barry and Helen are high-level scientists in a research facility at a prestigious university. "Yes, we definitely debate science over the dinner table," said Barry. "But not about what we do at work, we agree not to take that home. We talk about the mathematics of how the bath water drains, or how the molecules behave in a roast cooking in the oven—stuff like that. It makes us incredibly close."

The problems of merging two high-powered academic careers has been examined by Londa Schiebinger (and her colleagues) of Stanford University in a study of faculty members at research universities. Thirty-six percent of 9,043 full-time academic faculty at 13 research universities reported having an academic partner. One problem of two academics in love is being able to work in the same university, which administrations are now making easier so as to attract and maintain valuable faculty.[15]

Some of the couples in our interviews reported having problems with saving face, being competitive with each other in their luster, not being able to relax/deal with down time, and resisting being dependent on each other, even in a natural way. Lanie and Don are partners in an internal medicine practice, a second marriage of two high-profile professionals. Said Lanie, *The worst is when we go to our country place. We don't take our Blackberries. We will go from playing croquet to a class at a farm in fruit canning to doing the Sunday crossword puzzle to making love, and for a 24-hour period I am only with "Don the high achiever." We're both used to being the authorities and being "on" and I'm often just as guilty, sort of egging him on: I'll find myself competing with my husband about the pace on the treadmill . . . Harold, are you still at 5.0?*

Having a shared business or practice confers economic and practical advantages to a couple, so what do they have to learn? It isn't as simple as taking a detective story and a glass of iced tea and lying in the hammock. "Relaxing" for the high-powered careerist couple is an issue that comes up often. Relationship counselor Leigh Cousins told us how an ambitious couple can sort this out:[16]

> If they were laid-back types, would we expect them to go on vacation and morph into aggressive go-getters? Then why would we expect the high-powered people to "relax" when on vacation?
>
> Relaxation is a state of mind. Different people relax in different ways. Some people love to lie on the beach all day and other people go nuts with that sort of inactivity; they might prefer to sail, play volleyball, wash the car, read, or watch TV!
>
> Often a spouse is really complaining about lack of intimacy. During the usual hectic blur of life we aren't as connected with our wives or husbands as we would like . . . we hope that during vacation there will be more time and opportunity for intimacy, but then, the busy pace keeps up and the intimacy doesn't happen.
>
> In general, I think high-powered careerists need to come to change their expectations. They're aggressive, competitive people, and this is part of their personalities, not something they can turn on and off. They might do best to look for snippets of down time and intimate time; a quiet, intimate hour here and there . . . instead of expecting a vacation to bring out a whole new side of their partner. Would we really want that, anyway? I would be unnerved if my man became a completely different person when we're on vacation. I rely on him to be fundamentally himself, with the same charms, same quirks, just a little bit mellower and tanner. I go on vacation to have more time with the same man I love, not to see him, or me, change into someone else.
>
> Also, the woman who eggs her husband on . . . she's probably upset with herself. She's not so much asking for intimacy and relaxation, she's trying to work on her own conflicted feelings. She's provoking him, for whatever reason. A woman who really wants relaxation doesn't challenge her husband on the treadmill.

FLEXIBILITY

While being flexible is a quality of all successful couples, it comes in especially handy for those who intertwine their work and love lives. Cate Blanchett, actress, and Andrew Upton, translator and playwright, met in 1996 when she was in his translation of Chekov's *The Seagull*. They married the next year and in the following 11 years had three sons. After working and living abroad for many years and feeling, to quote Upton, that if they stayed away from their country they would be "adrift," they moved back to Sydney.

Upton translated *Hedda Gabbler* for his wife to perform at the Sydney Theater Company in 2004. They discovered they liked collaborating artistically and became the dual heads of the company as a result. Fascinatingly, Blanchett and Upton shared the directing duties of a double bill of short plays by David Mamet in 2006. The husband directed one half of the evening, and the wife the other, with the same set of actors appearing in both plays.

Being a support for the partner is something many working couples describe as a natural result of working together. The marriage of Tom Hanks and Rita Wilson illustrates this. Tom was an assistant to Rita while she produced *My Big Fat Greek Wedding*, and she coached him on his Balkan accent in *The Terminal*. Kevin Bacon and Kyra Sedgwick have worked on films together, and he has directed some of the episodes of her TV show, *The Closer*. (Both these couples met, fell in love at work, and married three years later).

RESOLVING CONFLICT

Couples who work together can benefit from an array of qualities—accepting criticism, accepting disparate work styles (e.g., working in spurts versus methodically), and resolving conflict. The couples we interviewed spoke of fighting, fury, and periods of discord. They spoke of the importance of not attacking their partner and keeping their disagreements impersonal. They knew how to have a loose enough disagreement that the tension level was not high. They valued each other over the project or the business. They were indispensible to each other. As a groundbreaking self-help book, *Intimate Enemies*, pointed out long ago, you can fight fair and both can win.[17]

Blanchett and Upton revealed their respective tempers in an interview in which Blanchett said, *We are each other's most constructive critic.* Upton agreed: *It's being able to honestly say, "Oh, I really failed; that really didn't work!"* At the theater where they are co-directors, they share a desk and a computer. Their clarity about keeping the communication channels open is evident in this remark by Upton: *We're trying to work out how to job-share while maintaining good communication within the company, so I don't end up with half the information and Cate ends up with the other half.*

TAKING TIME TO PLAY

Office lovers who become business partners don't forget what drew them to each other: fun. They are not constantly worrying over annual evaluations or goals. Being playful, Johan Huizinga suggested in *Homo Ludens*, is a prerequisite for progress in civilization. He wrote, "Not being 'ordinary' life, play stands outside the immediate satisfaction of wants and appetites, indeed it interrupts the appetitive process. It interpolates itself as a temporary activity satisfying in itself and ending there . . . as an intermezzo, an interlude in our daily lives."[18] This does not mean that work is a constant picnic, but a relaxed atmosphere certainly eases the tensions of daily life. There is an organic connection between home and work, which is uncommon.

SEPARATE SPACES

Everyone needs an environment that features individual private space. Marcus met Charlene when he designed a patio addition for the restaurant her parents owned. Marcus loved being part of his wife's big Italian family—for a while. *By the first anniversary, there was too much togetherness,* he said. *They got more and more pushy about our having a baby. Charlene was getting her business degree and still working as a hostess at night to please her parents, and I helped out on weekends at the bar to please them and also to protect Charlene from her relatives' jibes about the fact we didn't have a kid.*

We separated and lived apart for the next three years, developing as people in our grown-up lives. That stopped the push to have a baby, and then we slept together on the sly and she got pregnant, so I moved back in. Charlene persuaded me to open a café with her in a resort town we both liked. In a way, we have reinvented ourselves on their same model, because we are together 24 hours a day and we enjoy it.

BEING IN BUSINESS/WORKING WITH YOUR LOVER: THE MAN'S VIEW

So how do "men" view working with their lover?

1. Men Enjoy the Companionship of a True Friend in Business. Men are more inclined than are women to feel lonely when unattached. In one study of 377 respondents, 25.9 percent of the men compared to 16.7 percent of the women reported feeling a "deep sense of loneliness."[19] Similarly, in another study,[20] the researcher found that one-quarter of

386 adult men reported that they did not have enough friends. Possible reasons were homophobia, a lack of role models, a fear of being vulnerable, and competition between men. Regardless of the reason, the result is the same. To have a true friend and to be in business with this friend/lover is a godsend for men. One of the men whom we interviewed, who is in business with his wife, said, *I'm not typical. My wife and I are friends and really enjoy working and being together.* (This man may be more typical than he knows.)

2. Men Are More Burdened by Business Than Are Women. One of the burdens of being socialized as a male in U.S. society is to feel the onus of responsibility to earn money and to make the business a success. They can't "turn it off." Indeed, men equate their identify with their occupational role. In a study on men and taking time off from work, one researcher[21] found that men were much less likely to do so. They cited fear that doing so would affect their job or career performance evaluation. Women, on the other hand, were much more likely to use all of their vacation time.

3. Men Are More Profit-Focused Than Are Women. Men are traditionally socialized to be providers, so this translates into ensuring that meat (in the case of the hunter) or money (in the case of today's male) is available. If an activity does not generate income, he questions its utility. Meanwhile, his partner may be more service- or relationship-focused and care less about the bottom line.

4. Men Vary in Their View. Men are like cars—there are different types. Some are controlling and condescending. Others are cooperative, negotiating, and egalitarian. In business, some men will prefer that the woman "run" the business while others will want to push her out of the way.

BEING IN BUSINESS/WORKING WITH YOUR LOVER: THE WOMAN'S VIEW

How do women view working with their lovers?

Relationship is the matrix of a woman's thinking, so she will sense a problem related to how she and her mate treat each other before the man will. We try to not jump with alarm, because we have lives—we are not relationship obsessed. Still, if we do feel it's off kilter we are going to find ways to show the man, whose "feeling" side is likely to be shut down when he works.

Whereas a man tends to be off/on—either consumed by work, or exercising his talent for guy friendship (often, playing sports or engaging in technical talk spliced with personal remarks), women tend to be living the work and love and home as a totality—with the dimensions interpenetrating. Men will work hard with a payoff of sex at the end of the day, while the woman wants "the kiss on the brow during the day." Said a young mother who works part-time with her husband, "Running our business, my children's needs, loving my husband—for me each of these parts of my life is watered down by the others."

In the military, to get something done, some need to know what's going on. Information is handed out on a need-to-know basis. Women said that men were conversational with friends or family, but when they worked often operated on this need-to-know basis, to the point of excluding the woman from what she should be apprised of. The women we interviewed saw themselves as more transparent. Having different communication styles was a topic to work out through communicating about it.

Men were perceived by women as more visionary and less adept at day-to-day business. Women did not see themselves as relegated to secretary, but seemed to feel empowered by what they could do, and do in balance (these were all successful working couples). Said one woman who has been a software consultant with her husband for 20 years, *He's like those drivers that weave in and out, and figure they can avoid a collision by keeping up a velocity 10 miles faster than the flow of traffic. He speeds by and I go through with the tasks of the day.*

A few women felt that the access to a sexual partner anytime was ideal, but more women spoke of keeping sexual fires burning as a challenge. Said one physician, *I am a strong woman, and men have thought that that means I want to call the shots in bed—i.e., be assertive. But as a strong woman, I want relief from being in charge. I love to be asked. I don't want to have to look over and see that he has an erection at four in the morning and take advantage of it. That's not a turn-on. I lie back and let my husband take charge and I love it.*

Some people, regardless of gender, turn work off and don't think about it; others want to mull over the business during off-hours, and are surprised that even the ambitious mate won't discuss their enterprise when they are not working. Some women wish they could compartmentalize better, e.g., "I envy my husband that he can enter the studio without an idea in his head." On the other hand, there are men who will bring their cell phones on vacation so they can make work calls between tennis sets, or while they fish. In any case, women concurred they felt their husbands didn't want to be interrupted with either quibbles or bright thoughts; said the wife in a business that installs solar heating, "He'll say 'This isn't urgent, is it?' before I even begin."

Women seem more apt to be aware of getting respect, of being heard. It's central for women because they have been slated to the inferior position in worldly matters by tradition. "With respect comes the ability to listen," said one woman who has an office supply store with her husband. *It doesn't matter if he is full time and I'm part-time, or who knows more about this aspect of the business or the other, in all cases, respect and the ability to listen makes a difference. Even when we disagree on something, being able to understand why the other person thinks something allows for acceptance.*

In regard to working together, men and women agree on three points:

1. That being exhausted from hard work is a factor that hasn't hurt their relationship;
2. That working together is a gradual learning to adapt over the years— "we make adjustments as we go along, like the course corrections of a boat," said one male engineer;
3. That with each gravitating to what he or she does best, the harmony they have achieved is essential, if not visible to outsiders.

Whether they work together all the time, or, as often happens, the man works fulltime and the woman manages the home and works on the business part-time, when they speak about their business the personal pronoun to each other and to clients/others is "us" and "we."

National Public Radio's Colin McEnroe described why he liked his job—that he was putting his energies into what he was passionate about and was meant to do. "It uses everything I've got—my brain and my voice, and I can be funny. At the end of the day, you feel used up in a pleasant way, sucked dry, and you say 'Oh I let it all on the playing field today.' "[22]

The relationship should be able to survive the work, for grownups do not give their hearts on a temporary basis. Perhaps the most illustrious twentieth-century American woman, anthropologist Margaret Mead, looked objectively at her own marriages. Her first husband was Luther Cressman, preparing for the ministry, and they divorced over the faith issue. Mead's only quarrel with him over the divorce was that he didn't want her to disclose that he was already engaged before the divorce was settled. Reo Fortune, a New Zealander whom she met aboard a ship from Samoa, was a fantastic work partner— for two years. They wrote all day and conversed into the night. Reo wanted careerist Margaret to keep house when they came to New York City to live, but she said that he was rankled being the husband of a celebrity (and she had to make all the adjustments). Then when Mead was coming up with a new theory of the relation between culture, personality, and sex, with Reo and Gregory Bateson (an English anthropologist), she fell in love with the latter, who was more sympathetic with her ideas. The last marriage, which took place when Gregory was 31 and Margaret was 35, endured, but there is no doubt that Mead put work first. She was a pioneer in her lifestyle as well as her field; she faced with pluck the complications in her marriages due to (certainly in part) changes in gender roles. For instance, she joked in her autobiography that her father was "always amused, although at times a little embarrassed, by his exotic sons-in-law."[23] But we can see in her various marriages what was very successful (intense working relationship) and what was not (being consumed by one's work to the point where nothing else matters).

Couples who work together seem to smile brightly in tandem, as though they had a "secret asset." Many couples surely do not make it: working together can aggravate their incompatibility, and make tempers flare. But if the couple can finesse it, they are like beginning potters: their first pots fly off the wheel, but then they master the technique, They end up with full cooperation and a lot more "quality time" than most couples know.

16

If the Office Romance Ends

If I go there will be trouble, if I stay there will be double.

The Clash

With regard to break ups, heartaches, and the dismal aftermath, "work" is not that different from "life." The workplace is just a unique context for both opportunities and hazards. Work is a wonderful way to meet someone special to love. But there is a downside: what happens when it doesn't work out and yet you both still work there?

FORESIGHT

If possible, be the one to call it off if you see the end coming; we can always keep our cool better as the person who ends the relationship. Most often, the person who initiates the breakup will experience an easier and quicker recovery than the one given the boot. There is time ahead to process the end and prepare for the fall. Love is never easy to end, but it's easier if you jump than if you are pushed.

Extricating yourself is like pressing forward through brambles. You are the one who has to say that you think it is best that you not see each other any more, that you cancel the trip the two of you had planned to Mexico, and that you delete his or her number from your cell phone. You must confront the sadness and feel the pain. If you are the injured party, the pain can take you to your knees.

THE TALK

According to *The Tale of Genji* (written in the year 1,000 AD by Lady Murasaki),[1] the greatest skill in male-female relations is being able to conclude an affair gracefully. Don't say more than you mean. Have a calm talk away from work about not seeing each other, and how you'll behave together, since both of you want to minimize the office fallout.

The talk includes:

1. Taking responsibility. Don't blame; rather take responsibility for the end: You need "to spend some time apart." Your partner will likely translate "the end," which is accurate and what you intend.
2. Avoiding mudslinging. Keep your guns in their holsters; nothing is to be gained by name-calling. Credit yourself for having found the other person desirable in the first place.
3. Taking the hit. If you are the person being terminated, appreciate that you are hearing it straight up, and that you're not left to wonder why the phone has stopped ringing. You are going to hear that the relationship held meaning for the other person—believe it and take the renewed self-regard that will refract into your overall understanding later.
4. Looking, not touching. Ending a relationship rarely calls for a warm hug . . . that is likely to confuse both of you. Smile with your eyes to show affection if you will, and use a gentle tone of voice, but no touching—that ignites.

FALLOUT AT THE OFFICE

After you have split up, the best attitude at work is to live on automatic pilot and to save your confusion, misery for off-work hours. Crucially, don't argue with the person. If you attack openly, the recriminations swarm like angry bees from a beehive. Stay away—just get through the day.

Don't expect it to be quick and easy. The sense of personal loss may assail the distraught injured party at erratic moments throughout the day. One woman said that, when she went down a staircase she gripped with all her might, fearing that she would lose her step and tumble down. Another interviewee recalled, "I would be in a meeting and my eyes would well up with tears (which I hid as best I could) if someone said something about what they were doing with family or friends on the weekend." Still other persons with whom we talked spoke of physical disequilibrium, being "stunned," trembling, and so forth. And there are others who knew the end was coming and feel glad that it is over. Meanwhile, the protocol is business as usual.

AFTER FIVE

At quitting time, the former lovers will leave the office (not together or to meet later) and will feel a sense of personal loss. The unique attributes of the now former intimate, and the good times once had, may come to one's mind. "Things would have been different had I done this or that, my life will not be the same. . . ." The grieving, put on hold during the day, may overwhelm one's thoughts.

Since everybody who loves goes through heartache, the desolate emotions are familiar. The end of love with someone we knew intimately may attack our very being. While the pain and suffering can vanish in a weekend if the end came after a brief affair, getting over an intense love affair can take 12 to 18 months (with follow-up quakes when there is a stimulus to remind us of the breakup). Eventually we recover and move on.

SOME STRATEGIES TO HELP WITH THE RECOVERY

April, one of the women we interviewed, knew when she waved goodbye to her co-worker, and left the flower farm where she was in charge of mail orders, that she was in for a rough time. The owner had told her he was going back to his wife. That was his house on the hill above the gardens, which she saw as she walked out of the building to her car.

I tried to keep my spirits up, but I was devastated. There was no future, only the terrible present. What I did seems comical as I recount it but at the time it was like battening down the hatches . . . On the way home I picked up food at a takeout restaurant, so somebody else would be feeding me until I got my bearings. I also bought banana split ice cream, a spicy romance, a cheap diary, and bubble bath at the drugstore. Then I went home, took a bath with bubbles a foot high, and crawled under a comforter. I think I was tucking myself in like a child, because once I got into bed with my cell phone (and my cat), I absolutely would not get up again. I never wrote more than a few paragraphs in the diary but I liked having it there. I had the total breakup kit, and I needed it!

April confessed that she repeated these proceedings "because they worked" day after day. *I had to be cool and collected while I was at work at the flower farm. I was plotting how to get another job, but I didn't want to blow up after three years there.* April created structure for herself, scripted herself at work, and stuck to her recovery plan.

Another post-breakup strategy that people found helpful was putting somebody else in charge of you—a mother, sibling or friend. They bring you food or invite you to sleep over, so you are surrounded by people who are not in emotional straits, and with whom you can debrief in a way you cannot at the office.

If your biological clock is seriously disordered by the reversal in love, it's time to join the yoga class at the gym. Exercise will reduce your stress, so get to it.[2] Some report that yoga improves one's sense of well-being and stress-related symptoms.[3]

Another strategy is to be aware of the roadmap of grief—and ending a love relationship involves grief. Elizabeth Kubler-Ross delineated five stages of grief (denial, anger, bargaining—"Let me just get through the next month"—depression, and acceptance), a model that is commonly taught in medical schools today.[4] However, the stages are not linear and neat, as she pointed out. A person can experience the stages all in a day, or out of order, as well as over a long time.

Still another strategy is not to look away when you see the person at the office. After awhile you will begin to see the person differently. One woman we interviewed who recounted her office romance breakup said, "It was catastrophic at the early stage to see him, but then I got kind of a reality check, where I didn't fantasize about this fabulous star-crossed person lost to me forever." A man who proposed to a fellow teacher at a school, and had to accept that she had never returned his feelings, said similarly that "seeing her frequently as I did seemed to stir the ashes so my rational brain could stamp out the fire."

Coreen, a musician in New York state, said, *Before my marriage I had several crushes on people who played in the same orchestras I did—I seemed to latch onto the string section! I learned over the years, once the initial pain has passed, to tell myself, "To hell with it." Then it fades and it becomes a non-issue.*

To deal with this initial pain, Coreen advised, *the best route is to feel the pain as intensely as possible—really work on getting into it. Each time it seems to return, feel it intensely again like a piece of music. Do this as often as necessary. I think that to try to avoid the pain ultimately makes the pain worse, more insidious and pervasive, and, of course that makes it hang around longer, sometimes much longer.* Lay people call this "facing your fears"; psychologists call this "implosion." Whatever you call it, exposure reduces the emotional pain over time.

VENGEANCE IS A BOOMERANG

Invariably, being vengeful is a losing tactic causing more unhappiness, or, as Francis Bacon wrote in his pithy essay *Of Revenge*, "This is certain, that a man that studieth revenge keeps his own wounds green, which otherwise would heal and do well."[5]

Tina, a publicist, was congratulated by her girlfriends when she tore everything off the messy desk of an associate who had jilted her, *but it was a moment's satisfaction with a fallout that wasn't worth it. It was okay to dress him down when we raked things over, I had to do that, but flailing around the office, casting things on the floor was absurd. I wish I hadn't.*

WORST-CASE SCENARIO

In the event that one of the two parties declares that he or she was coerced, and sues for sexual harassment, a poison is released that affects each of them. This scenario is discussed in Chapter 17. A predictor of how someone will behave if "discarded" by a sexual partner may be whether the person was prone to litigation in his or her past, and how bellicose he or she is.

WHY YOU DON'T BURN YOUR BRIDGES

Closure is required when you break up with a lover: that's why you have "the talk," and why you don't let yourself phone and/or text at 3 a.m. But when the romance is in the office, there is a special twist: if you treat the person respectfully, even if he or she is/seems to be a cur at the time, you may have an ally for life.

Cyril's business involves hooking up big celebrities with big endorsements. He usually employs just one assistant, and there is a fairly rapid turnover when that person goes on to bigger and better things. After his divorce, he wined, dined, and had an affair with the next assistant he hired, a talented MBA, Nancy. Cyril was in his mid-forties and Nancy was 23. Cyril thought he was a good guy to break it off after a lot of locked eyes and candlelight suppers and only one interlude in bed.

Cyril was sincere that Nancy was too young, and it felt too serious with her, and he wanted her to have a "big, big life" (evolve as he sensed she would, and believed one ought). Nancy recognized that in his mind he could date and have a fling with someone nearer his age more safely. She recalls that, *I had a strong intuition that it wasn't over, that we had an intimate link that would reassert in some positive way.* She found another job. Some years later, she and Cyril formed a company together, to their mutual success. They hadn't forseen this, but as it turnsout, trusted each other on a deeper level because of how each weathered the romance that was not meant to be.

If a person stays in the company or even the career, a measure of diplomacy can be like the stitch in time saves nine. Dorothy broke up with her boyfriend at a small law firm where she worked. *He thanked me for convincing him to get a new job* she said. *He didn't have to remember how I kept his shirt in my closet for a year, or burned the photos of him in a little pyre, because he didn't know that embarrassing stuff. The love, after all, had been mine, not his, and because I had the luck or wisdom to think of it that way, it was no problem to work with him, even though I had been very disappointed when his feelings proved inconstant.*

RISKS TO THE COMPANY

Do you care? You probably do if you stayed long enough to have formed this attachment—you may care about your reference letter, if nothing else! Don't make people you work with take sides. This isn't a boxing match. If people work with you, they have allegiance to each of you. Plus, it is sometimes the pattern that men want to side with men and women want to side with women. This has the potential to cause an unfriendly and counterproductive tangle.

Besides sexual harassment charges, businesses are sometimes ruined by disputes between ex-romantic partners. Often the scar is so deep that the couple is unable to work together after they call it quits. A partnership in love and business successful enough to create/carry on a viable business will usually be derailed if the relationship ends. The Mia Farrow-Woody Allen split ended her appearance in subsequent Allen movies.

Women today are wise when it comes to business. Penny and her professor husband Dick bought a thriving fuel company at a good price. Ten years later, when Dick decided he not only wished to be richer but to have a younger woman, and left Penny, she had her wits about her. Instead of recriminations, she focused on securing the business for herself and her sons. Now grown up, they have developed and run it with her.

HEAL THYSELF

When the relationship ends, focus on getting yourself back on track, rather than getting back at your partner. The grave mistake that people make, said one of our respondents (also a relationship counselor), is that they look outward instead of inward. *People need to focus on their own development. Young women in particular should work on their finances and career, independence (all aspects), emotional stability, education, social connection, and community involvement. And a few rounds of therapy may be helpful—especially if they've been single for a while and don't want to be, or had one train-wreck relationship after another. These things aren't about chance or bad luck; this is how you are doing something. You need to look at that.*

The central theme of this chapter is to regard the end of an office romance like the end of a movie. It's time to get up and move on. Do whatever you can to be gracious, polite, and forgiving, and then move forward. Like the last line of the Eagles classic rock song "Wasted," which speaks to the end of an intense love affair: "It wasn't wasted at all." If the office romance ends, you loved, you learned, move on.

17

Office Romance Policies and Sexual Harassment

Whether they publish a dating policy or don't publish a dating policy—
somebody is going to get screwed.
                              Lucy Johnson, Retired State Employee

There are some people who say no matter how attracted they are to
someone, "I'm not going to pursue the relationship if we work in the
same firm." The pitfall they fear is that "if it doesn't work out, we'll
have to see each other day after day." And even worse, there will be
a sexual harassment suit. But an office romance is easy to develop if
one works long hours, works weekends, and travels extensively.
Indeed, individuals are biologically wired for attractions to occur even
if one is pair-bonded and has no intention to pursue another relationship. In addition, many people will be more disposed to become
involved with someone at work than they would online since the person is "there" and is a "known."

While love is a private matter, 9 to 5 romance becomes a public matter when it has the potential to affect the organization that employs the
lovers. The primary concern of the employer is economic: Will love
between employees cause a loss of productivity? Probably not.
Indeed, 9 percent of the respondents in our Internet Office Romance
Survey reported that their office romance was associated with an
increase in their productivity (73% said that it made no difference).
A sexual harassment suit is also unlikely. Less than 3 percent of
respondents in our survey reported filing such a claim. Since the
potential for something to go wrong with romance in the workforce
is minimal, three-fourths of companies have no written policy about

dating a co-worker.[1] In a survey of the American Management Association, 70 percent of managers in their thirties and forties said that it was okay for employees to date (66% of managers in their fifties and sixties agree).[2]

DOES A COMPANY HAVE THE RIGHT TO RESTRICT OFFICE ROMANCE?

Should a company have the right to restrict a love relationship that begins to spark during the workday? It depends on whom you ask. Attorney Bob Gregg of the Boardman law firm of Madison, Wisconsin, noted that sexual harassment lawyers warn that if there is a policy in place that states that co-workers are to stay clear of each other, that will provide a defense in the event that one of the lovers becomes a stalker, or if a sexual harassment suit is filed. Some civil rights advocates say that such policies violate personal rights, and are unlawful.[3]

TYPES OF POLICIES RELATED TO OFFICE ROMANCE

There are at least four types of policies related to office romances:[4]

1. No Fraternization. This policy prohibits all romantic advances, overtures, and relationships by anyone toward anyone in the company. Wal-Mart has a no fraternization policy. It wants its employees focused on serving the customers, not romancing each other.
2. Power Model. This policy prohibits any romantic advances, overtures, and relationships by anyone whom a person in the company has authority over. Boss-secretary, and supervisor-supervisee relationships are the target of this policy. UPS uses this power model for romantic relationships between managers/supervisors and employees. Some companies also exclude anyone at a higher rank becoming involved with anyone of a lower rank, even though that person is not directly being supervised.
3. No Extramarital. This policy prohibits anyone from being part of a relationship where one of the parties (or both) is married to someone else. The Air Force particularly takes a dim view of a married person having a romance with someone other than his or her spouse. Kelly Flinn was discharged from the U.S. Air Force in 1997 after being charged with adultery (sex with a man who was married to an enlisted female), fraternization, and lying.[5]

4. Consensual Relationships. This policy acknowledges that such relationships will develop, and asks only that the parties inform their immediate supervisor of any romantic relationship so that it can be confidentially verified that the relationship is "welcome/consensual." Some companies require the parties to sign a form that their relationship is consensual. The goal of this policy is to help ensure that a sexual harassment suit is not filed in the future. In reality, it is doubtful if most dating couples will acknowledge to their supervisor that they are seeing each other.

If you are fired from your job because of an office romance, you must prove that state laws protect your right to date. In many cases, state statutes indirectly protect dating, but it is left up to the court to interpret this.[6]

WHEN OFFICE ROMANCE BECOMES THE BUSINESS OF BUSINESS

Corporations become particularly anxious when workplace lovers occupy different hierarchical positions. A romance between a boss and a subordinate creates an issue for the corporation, since a potential exists for exploitation (the boss uses his power/status to get sex and then dumps the woman, resulting in her retaliation) or sexual harassment (this will be defined later in this chapter). If a lawsuit is filed, the cost in 2009 dollars to defend the lawsuit is $104,000 in legal fees, in addition to the unwanted negative publicity.[7] In addition, corporations feel that some overt office romances may look unprofessional, and set an undesirable tone for the workplace.[8]

In a study of romance in the workplace conducted by the Society for Human Resource Management, 80 percent of HR professionals and 60 percent of HR employees agreed that supervisors and subordinates should not become romantically involved.[9]

WHEN THERE IS SAME-SEX ATTRACTION

Due to a heterosexual societal bias, discussions of office romance usually assume that the lovers are heterosexual. This model does not capture lesbian love relationships, which are more often formed between equals. In a study of lesbian love relationships on the job, Dr. Schneider observed that the potential for exploitation and sexual harassment are minimized. In addition, the researcher found that lesbian lovers are more likely to remain friends when the love relationship is over.[10]

That firms are sensitive to gay issues was revealed in the 2001 French movie *The Closet*, which takes place when it was okay to be gay in the workplace. When the protagonist, a middle-range accountant with a loser personality in a large firm is fired, he ("Pignon" played by Daniel Auteuil) claims he's gay and the firm, afraid of a lawsuit and bad publicity not only restores his position, but promotes him.

SEXUAL HARASSMENT

The term "office romance" implies that both parties are in an emotionally intimate consensual relationship. But "sex in the office" has another connotation, referencing where there may be sexual exploitation and/or sexual harassment. The official policy of businesses in the United States is that sexual harassment is unacceptable, that employees are to be treated with respect and that sexual innuendos are off limits. Sexual harassment can cost the company money in employee turnover, lawsuits, and missed days at work.

Sexual Harassment Defined

The Equal Employment Opportunity Commission has defined sexual harassment and made it clear that it is a form of sex discrimination that violates Title VII of the Civil Rights Act of 1964. Sexual harassment (men are most often the perpetrator) is defined as unwelcome sexual advances (he puts his hand on your shoulder and leaves it there), requests for sexual favors ("how about a blow job in the copy room?"), or requests for out-of-office time ("how about meeting me for a drink after work?") which are tied to the person's work role. If the woman moves her shoulder or says "no" to the copy room suggestion or "no" to the drink invitation, and the boss retaliates by assigning her more work, giving her a bad evaluation, overlooking her for promotion/ salary increases, or firing her, sexual harassment has occurred. The most frequent target of sexual harassment is the financially vulnerable female working for a male who holds status and economic power over her.[11] While there are other categories of sexual harassment (women harassing men, men harassing men, and women harassing women), we will focus on the most typical.

Two General Types of Sexual Harassment

There are two overarching types of sexual harassment. The first is *hostile environment* sexual harassment, which refers to deliberate or repeated unwanted sexual comments or behaviors that affect one's performance at work or school. A female employee comes to work and is met by the boss, who asks her, "Get any over the weekend?" and stares at her breasts. He may even touch her new blouse and say "Nice." For the employee, the result is a fear of what he will do next. She is continually walking a tightrope of turning down his advances while maintaining her job. In our Internet Office Romance Survey, almost 20 percent (18.8%) of the respondents reported that they had experienced someone touching them at work that made them uncomfortable; almost 30 percent (29.8%) reported that they had experienced someone's saying something sexual to them at work that made them uncomfortable.

A second type of sexual harassment is *quid pro quo* (something for something) which means that if the female smiles when asked if she "got any?," meets the boss in the copy room, or has a drink after work, she can expect to be rewarded by keeping her job, being promoted, or getting a salary increase. Indeed, she is viewed as playing along (and often fears not doing so).

Two of the most unwanted sexual harassment workplace behaviors are those of unwanted touching and the invasion of personal space. Others include:

- Rumoring—spreading sexual gossip behind a target's back
- Sexual graffiti or material placed on a target's desk
- Personal questions
- Sexual posturing
- Pressure for dates or relationships

Regardless of the sexual harassment behavior, the victim does not have to be the person harassed but could be anyone affected by the offensive conduct. For example, let's say you are not harassed by your boss, but your co-worker is and you feel her pain; this is sexual harassment since you are subjected to this context.

Unlawful sexual harassment may occur without economic injury to or the discharge (firing) of the victim. Hence, even though you did not play along and still got a raise, you are a victim of sexual harassment since you were put in a hostile environment. The primary factor that must be present is that the harasser's conduct was unwelcome and that you felt pressure to endure it.

Whatever the specifics of the sexual harassment, the workplace becomes highly aversive, as revealed by one of the young females we interviewed who works for a large insurance agency. Faye summarized the agency where she has been employed for two years. *There is about a 60/40 mix of women to men [60% women]. The woman who is the head administrator is said to have had the boss's baby . . . his wife also works with us and she also had his baby. I know he has dated at least one other woman in the office, and he currently has a lawsuit pending with a staff member who still works with us. She had her lawyers come in and basically tell him that she couldn't be fired or mistreated, given her proof of his sexual harassment.*

Most of the time, he hits on girls and continues until they give in. He uses his power to manipulate women in the office. If his "prey" doesn't agree to his suggestions, he makes her life hell: He says things about her to other staff members, he tells lies (that the person is chronically late, for example) to his executive staff, and makes the uncooperative person a target. He is very persuasive and surrounds himself with weak people so that he can manipulate them into whatever situation he needs. Take his wife, for example: she believes everything he says, even though she hears the rumors in the office about him and other women, and has caught him being unfaithful in the past.

The women in the office feel as though they need to play along. This translates into not saying anything back to him, not telling the human resource person what is going on (because the HR person is best friends with the boss), and eventually quitting because of the stress of working there.

I have dodged being fired by not saying anything back to him. I also do my job so he cannot really fire me for anything job related. Most people quit, and some have tried to file a sexual harassment claim against him. The lawsuits were not successful since either the woman ran out of money, or there was a lack of evidence. The boss has lawyers on standby for this sort of thing.

Also, the boss does not usually fire people, because then they can draw unemployment benefits. Instead, he makes their lives a living hell until they quit.

People should be aware that regulations can be twisted against an innocent person by someone who wishes to inflict harm. Sometimes one may be innocent of any sexual harassment charges; if this is the case, that person should not suffer in silence. Andre was everybody's friend at the large health club where he worked. Then he was fired for alleged sexual harassment. Andre racked his brains to think whom he might have offended. His employer wasn't telling: the file was sealed in the personnel office.

An electrical engineer who had also trained Olympic athletes in East Europe, Andre was taking courses to prepare him for a civil engineering certification in the United States. Meanwhile, he was at the gym (and liked his work). When Andre was fired he was not going to bow down to anonymous accusers (especially since his father had been imprisoned without a trial under a Communist regime). Andre hired an attorney who easily procured Andre's file. He opened the file in the company of several people who went to the gym, so no one would suspect him of tampering with its contents. In that file, among the many letters of praise for Andre was one scrawled note that said, "I was at the water fountain and he came over and said I lost weight and touched my upper arm."

Guilty as charged! Now Andre recalled complimenting a heavyset, middle-aged woman on the results of her diet and exercise program, and giving her a pat of encouragement. That she had a crush on him was general knowledge, although he was unaware of it. Eventually Andre was told by personnel they had made an error, the woman who made the complaint quit the club, and Andre's lawyer, a client of the health club who had taken up Andre's cause, refused to accept payment from Andre for legal services. Andrew held his head high and found new employment.

TOLERANCE VARIES BY THE CULTURE OF THE CAREER/JOB/CONTEXT

We interviewed a Wall Street attorney in his fifties. He observed that while today there is less teasing, sexual innuendo, and banter than there was 20 years ago, there are *some industries which remain more animal houses than others—Wall Street being one of them. Things are said on the traditional floor that are potentially actionable, but women there develop a thick skin. They learn quickly it's not worth the hassle and it's advantageous to be one of the boys. Short of a physical attack, a female on Wall Street is going to pay no attention to a sexist comment or joke, or even a hand placed on her. She will explain, "I don't want to be known as a bitch."*

Sometimes an employee might try to use the law to her advantage. The attorney gave this example: In the mid-1990s, "at the height of sexual harassment lawsuits" a European woman was out at a bar with fellow attorneys, all in their mid-twenties. *It was ten at night, and one guy was a little tipsy. He said, "Hey babe," and lightly touched her arm. She smiled in a tight-lipped fashion, and a week later complained to Human Resources that she had been sexually harassed.*

I was the immediate boss of both of them. My job was to investigate the behavior and make a judgment. I talked with both separately and with witnesses, and concluded that it was an innocent gesture, not a sexual come-on.

I told the man who was accused, "You were on the line but it doesn't rise to sexual harassment." He apologized to her. He really didn't think he'd done anything intentionally harassing. He wasn't being difficult when he apologized—it wasn't a stubborn, "to hell with her" kind of thing.

However, the woman said his apology was not acceptable. She went to HR, who also said the incident didn't rise to sexual harassment. HR said to drop it. The woman then sued the firm, and the case went to trial. She lost: the jury said it was not sexual harassment. The woman left the firm of her own accord before the trial and she and her husband left the U.S. permanently shortly after that. I came to the conclusion that she was scamming the system to get a financial settlement.

EXTENT AND CONTEXTS OF SEXUAL HARASSMENT

About half of all working women in the United States are affected by sexual harassment.[12] In terms of sexual harassment in different professions, 88 percent of female nurses, 70 percent of female office workers, 64 percent of women in the U.S. military, and 51 percent of female family practice resident physicians report having been sexually harassed.[13] Although sexual harassment of men does occur, it is less common because men have greater power in society. Indeed, sexual harassment is often directed toward young, unmarried women in traditionally all-male organizations. Women in the military reserve are particular targets of sexual harassment, with 60 percent reporting such harassment (the percent includes sexual assault during service). Branches with the highest and lowest percentages of harassment charges during their service are the Navy, at 57.1 percent, and the Marines at 75 percent.[14]

Gay and lesbian individuals are also vulnerable to sexual harassment in the workplace. Based on a study of more than 2,000 adult workers in the United States, 41 percent of the gay and lesbian workers reported facing some form of hostility or harassment on the job. Almost 1 in 10 of the gay or lesbian workers stated that he or she had been fired or dismissed unfairly from a previous job, or pressured to quit a job, because of his or her sexual orientation.[15]

WHY MEN SEXUALLY HARASS WOMEN

In our Internet Office Romance Survey, 28 percent of the respondents agreed that "men exploit women sexually in the workplace." Some explanations for sexual harassment follow:[16]

1. Male Sex Drive. Men are driven to have sex with women and use sexual harassment as a means to gain compliance/sexual access to more women.
2. Male Dominance in Society. Men typically occupy higher status positions in organizations, which reflect male social and political dominance in the larger society.
3. Job Requirements. The expectations of some jobs may encourage sexual harassment. For example, there may be personal appearance requirements for women, which include that they wear dress shoes, a skirt—that they be professionally dressed. There may also be requirements for travel or working behind closed doors. The result is that women are expected to be beautiful and feminine and travel/work with powerful men who affect their jobs.

There are times when sex on the job is not a problem. For example, when there is consensual agreement so that the respective parties feel all is fair in what they are giving and getting. Two women we interviewed spoke of a clear-eyed trade with a boss of sex for special privileges. Both were over 40, and looking back at a time when they were unpartnered in their thirties. Said Rainey, *I got a job in PR. It was just my boss and me on the West Coast, and his business partner in the East. He told me that I could take off when I had to, for doctor's appointments or parent-teacher conferences. I'd been there a year when he separated from his wife. One day he asked me to have sex with him to calm him down before a client went on national TV. I said I needed something too—an arrangement where I did the work on my own schedule. With the limo waiting downstairs to take him to the station, I performed oral sex on him. From then on when he was antsy he would pull his chair out from his desk and I did what he wanted me to. Honestly I felt less guilty about the sex than I had about leaving early or going out in the middle of the day to do what I needed to as a single mother. This went on for a year, until I moved back with my parents. My boss actually treated me fairly and professionally, exclusive of this weird and customary sexual act.*

The other woman who serviced a boss in a job she desperately needed as a single mother knew from the interview that the boss was looking for an employee/mistress. *In retrospect, I am amazed I had the gall. The situation went on for four years. Nobody would ever have known, except that when I started to have intercourse with someone else, he asked why I didn't have curtains in my bedroom. I said it was a northern exposure, and that I wanted all the light . . . Besides, no man ever spent the night. He picked up on that right away. "You have been divorced five years and I'm the first man to spend the night?" He put two and two together and figured out that I'd been carrying on with my boss. "He's not that bad and you do*

what you have to," I said, and Stan left it at that. He felt as I did, that our sex-
ual pasts were water under the bridge. Sometimes men don't want to know
the details.

CONDITIONS OF SEXUAL HARASSMENT

Four conditions must be met for sexual harassment to occur:[17]

1. Motivation to harass. Sex, power, and control are among the motives for sexual harassment. Some men are sadistic, in that they get pleasure out of manipulating an economically destitute women who can't afford to lose her job or quit, so she puts up with the harassment.
2. Overcoming internal inhibitions that might suppress harassment. Most men would like to have sex with women in the office and elsewhere. In most cases, common sense, judgment, character, and integrity over-rule these libidinous thoughts so that the man is polite and respectful. Men who harass with wild abandon have lost their way—they don't care whom they denigrate and don't care what others think of their behavior. Alcohol or other drugs, a history of "successful" harassment, and being unhappy in one's life and relationships are all associated with sexual harassment.
3. Overcoming external inhibitions. Noted earlier was the example of the office employee whose boss had "his lawyers on standby" to handle sexual harassment complaints. Men who harasse feel insulated from retaliation, so they do not fear the consequences of being sexually aggressive. It is a despicable situation when lawyers are hired to protect men who exploit women who need a job and to be respected while putting in a day's work.
4. Overcoming victim resistance. Most women abhor sexual harassment and run from it. The modus operandi of the harasser is basically to wear the woman down by his consistent and relentless pursuit. If the woman is economically depressed that may tempt her to give in. Or she may quit.

POLICIES DESIGNED TO REGULATE SEXUAL HARASSMENT

To help reduce sexual harassment in the workplace, the Equal Employment Opportunity Commission (EEOC) of the federal government, major companies, and academic institutions have developed sexual harassment policies. The formal goals of these policies are to go on record as being against sexual harassment, to discourage employees from engaging in sexually harassing behavior, and to provide a mechanism through which harassment victims can inform management. The informal goals are to provide the organization with guidelines for reacting to allegations of harassment, to protect the organization from being taken to court, and to reduce the chance of having to pay punitive damages if a lawsuit is filed. Organizations and schools also offer educational programs about sexual harassment and develop and distribute brochures and conduct training workshops. Increasingly, policies emphasize the rights of the harassed, the responsibility of the organization to prevent harassment, and the mechanisms for dealing with harassment should it occur.

Those who file sexual harassment suits may encounter empathy for their experiences, or they may discover that the full weight of the organization is being used against them. The institution may be willing and have the resources to launch a full-scale attack on the professional, personal, and sexual life of the complainant. In spite of the 3,000 military women serving in Iraq and Afghanistan who reported being sexually assaulted in 2008, the Pentagon estimates that 80 to 90 percent of sexual assaults are not reported. Reasons include the belief that nothing will be done, fear of ostracism, and further harassment. "A lot of my male colleagues believe that the only thing a general needs to worry about is whether he can win a war," says Congresswoman Loretta Sanchez of the Armed Services Committee.[18]

In effect, there is double victimization. Not only must the woman endure being sexually harassed at work (which may include sexual assault), if she complains and the case goes to court, she may find herself on the witness stand, being asked about her sex life. The goal of the defense attorney is to create the impression that this woman is a slut, has a history of sleeping with men, and came on to her boss to exploit his power/get a salary increase/promotion. The fact that none of these accusations are true is irrelevant—the goal of the defense attorney is to make pursuing a sexual harassment claim so aversive that she backs off and drops the suit. It is often the case that those who file sexual harassment complaints end up withdrawing them.[19]

Sexual Harassment in Educational Settings

The greatest amount of sexual harassment occurs not from faculty to students, but from students to faculty. In a study of 102 faculty and 359 college students at a large Midwestern university, more than half (53%) of the faculty reported having experienced at least one sexually harassing behavior from students; 63 percent of the students reported engaging in potentially sexually harassing behaviors at least once toward faculty members.[20] The students did not differ by gender in their likelihood of perpetrating sexual harassment. However, the women professors reported more unwanted sexual attention than did the men professors; and were also more bothered by such unwanted sexual attention.

Research on sexual harassment charges by students toward faculty has concluded that such cases involve vague definitions of what constitutes harassment, with faculty being denied proper hearings and being fired even if they have tenure.[21] In fact, sexual harassment charges provide administrators a way to fire faculty with tenure, something they might like to do but are typically precluded from doing. The faculty member who is accused of sexual harassment is often as good as convicted even before any testimony is heard.

CONSEQUENCES OF SEXUAL HARASSMENT FOR VICTIMS

Sexual harassment may be devastating for victims. Direct experiences with harassment can lead to a shattering of victims' core assumptions about the world and themselves, which, in turn, can result in considerable psychological distress. Victims complain of depression, anxiety, anger, fear, guilt, helplessness, sexual dysfunction, isolation from family/friends, and substance abuse.[22] Although not all sexually harassing events constitute a trauma, researchers are finding that nearly one-third of sexual harassment victims meet the symptom criteria for PTSD diagnosis.[23]

Sexual harassment may also become a "threat to an individual's resources by threatening financial resources . . . losses can occur in terms of lost job, lost status among coworkers, failure to gain a raise or promotion, lost interpersonal supports, and lost esteem regarding one's work."[24]

RESPONSES OF VICTIMS TO SEXUAL HARASSMENT

Employees who are targets or victims of sexual harassment most often typically ignore it. Unfortunately, ignoring harassment does not make it go away. Some women try to avoid the harasser by never being alone with him, asking for a transfer, or quitting the job. These indirect strategies are not very effective, and do nothing to deter the harasser from violating others.

Victims are not more blatant in their protests, since they fear retaliation if they do complain. In a sample of almost 3,000 women, almost 60 percent (57%) of those who had been harassed reported that they felt that their chances of promotions or pay raises would be hurt if they complained. As a result of feeling that they would experience limited gains from complaining, less than 15 percent of victims file formal sexual harassment complaints.[25]

CONFRONTING SOMEONE WHO SEXUALLY HARASSES YOU

Aside from ignoring or avoiding the sexual harasser, a victim has at least three choices: verbal, written, and institutional/legal action. The verbal choice consists of telling the harasser what behavior he or she is engaging in that creates discomfort and asking the person to stop. The victim could soften the accusation by saying something like, "You may not be aware that some of the things you say and do make me uncomfortable. . . . "Some harassers will respond with denial ("What are you talking about? I was just joking."); others will apologize and stop the behavior. When a full apology is offered, in which the offering party assumes full responsibility, the victim accepts and moves on.

If direct communication fails to terminate the harassment, a written statement of the concerns is the next level. Such a letter details the sexual harassment behaviors (with dates of occurrence) and includes a description of the consequences (personal distress, depression, sleeplessness). The letter should end with a statement of what the victim would like to happen in the future. For example, "I ask that our future interaction be formal and professional. This means do not touch me, tell any sexual jokes, or make any sexual references."

The letter should be sent immediately after it becomes clear that the offender did not take the verbal requests for change seriously. If the desired behavior is not forthcoming, the letter can be used as evidence of an attempt to alert the offender of the sexual harassment problem. Use of this evidence may be internal (inside the organization) or external (a formal complaint filed with the Equal Employment Opportunity Commission). Information for filing a complaint with the EEOC can be found by typing in "Sexual harassment" in the search feature of its website at http://www.eeoc.gov/. As noted earlier, in our Internet Office Romance Survey, less than 3 percent (2.6%) of the respondents reported filing a formal complaint of sexual harassment by someone at work. Throughout the U.S., about 14,000 complaints are submitted annually to the EEOC (85% are submitted by women).[26]

Unfortunately, women who take the direct approach to confront the harasser are at greater risk for experiencing adverse psychological and somatic symptoms than those who attempt to solve the problem indirectly. Although the direct approach is assertive, harassment victims who speak up often encounter reprisals, counterallegations, forced time off from work, and slander.[27] Although 97 percent of women at an elite military academy experienced sexual harassment during a six-month period (48 percent on a recurring basis), only 26 cases were reported in a five-year period. The primary reason that the women did not report the harassment is that they thought that nothing would be done, and that there would be negative consequences in the form of retaliation and isolation.[28]

A woman in an executive position in a New York law firm was asked if she had ever experienced sexual harassment. "I am sexually harassed every day," she said. Then she shrugged. "But I deal with it." Today a working woman (or man) does not have to suffer the slings and arrows of a boss gone wild alone. Going to court can be agonizing, but there is a superstructure of laws available to the employee who wants to challenge their employer.

SEXUAL HARASSMENT OF MEN

The term "sexual harassment" typically conjures up the image of the subordinate female employee as the victim of an outrageous boss who controls her job and her future in exchange for sexual favors. Or she, at least, is the target of sexual jokes, inappropriate touching, you name it. But some corporations feature women in positions of power, and men are expected to do their bidding. One such corporation is Jenny Craig, with a woman as chief executive of the over 4,000 employees—most of whom are women.

Eight of the men who had worked at the Jenny Craig weight loss centers in the Boston area charged the company with sex discrimination and sexual harassment, saying that "they were fired, denied promotion, or given unfavorable assignments because they were outsiders in a female-dominated corporate culture. . . . A few of them say they were taunted about their "tight buns" . . . one Jenny Craig plaintiff said that his female supervisor told him she dreamed of him naked."[29]

Indeed, advice by Dr. Marie McIntyre (workplace psychologist)[30] to both women and men in the workplace in regard to avoiding a sexual harassment suit is to be *vigilant about the potential for sexual harassment and to be very conscious about determining whether any advances are welcome. And if their partner has ended the relationship, they must stop pursuing it in any way. Continued pursuit could be viewed as harassment, especially if the person is a manager.*

OVERVIEW OF POLICY OPTIONS

The law provides a path for someone who has been sexually harassed. In June 1998, the U.S. Supreme Court held that an employer could be automatically liable for a supervisor's sexual harassment of a subordinate. The employee who feels that she has been denied opportunities in the workplace because she or he did not agree to become emotionally or sexually involved with a supervisor (or a fellow employee) may complain to the equal employment opportunity (EEO) officer. This action should result in an investigation.

While most companies/corporations look the other way at office romances, some have written policies that they hold their employees accountable to. The following is a review is these alternatives:

1. No Policy. Common sense rules and the company/corporation hope they don't get a sexual harassment suit. And they recognize they can be sued anyway.
2. No Dating Policy. Also known as antifraternization policies, this guideline is often hidden inside the antinepotism section. The State of Nevada has such a "nepotism/dating relationship" policy that *prohibits a classified employee from working under the immediate supervision or in direct line of authority of someone with whom he or she is having "a dating relationship" or a family member, including spouse, child, parent, aunt, uncle, niece, nephew, grandparent, grandchild, or first cousin of the same relation by marriage.... "Dating relationship" is defined as an intimate association primarily characterized by the expectation of affectional or sexual involvement. The term does not include a casual relationship or an ordinary association between personas in a business or social context.*[31]
3. Notification Policy. Employees are required to report their involvement in a romantic, consensual relationship with someone at work to the designated company representative (for example, your EEO officer). This policy helps protect the company if the romantic relationship goes sour and the person did not report the relationship.
4. Love contract. Also known as a consensual relationship agreement, a love contract is a document which states that a relationship exits and is voluntary/consensual, that the parties know of the sexual harassment

policy and how to report complaints, and identifies any expected behavior, such as refraining from displays of affection at work or retaliation if the relationship ends.

FIRST DAY AT WORK? A LEGAL PREP

Suppose it is your first day a work in Corporate America and you want to avoid the legal bus hitting you as you navigate the idea of an office romance. John Endicott, an attorney who has practiced in Texas, New York, and Connecticut, offers this advice:

When you agreed to begin your current job, your employer may have asked you to sign an agreement requiring you to notify your H.R. department in the event you have a dating or sexual relationship with an employee supervising you or whom you supervise.

Generally, the purpose of such a policy is to assure that the relationship involves mutual consent, rather than quid pro quo sexual harassment, where an employee's sexual submission to a supervisor's unwelcome advances is used as the basis for employment decisions.

But employers can also be legitimately concerned that employee morale may suffer if there is actual or perceived favoritism as a result of a dating relationship between you and someone with authority to affect your career. That is why some corporations' policies, as Washington, D.C., attorney Barbara Johnson recommends, also reserve the employer's right to "alter the reporting relationship of the parties involved, which may involve reassignment of either or both of the parties." So you could be sent to another division in another state for a dalliance.

One other scenario to be aware of: a number of courts have held that the married owner of a business may be within his or her right in terminating an actual, or even a would-be, employee paramour. In one case,[32] the fired employee merely "wrote notes of a sexual or intimate nature" to her boss, whose wife then found one of these notes in the company dumpster, pieced it together, and gave her husband an ultimatum: either the employee had to go or she would.

The workplace is a wonderful context in which to meet a romance partner and potential mate. But business is business, and lovers need to be aware of the legalities involved and mind their manners. In reality, workers can have it both ways. They can enjoy the romance ride and do their job. And one often enhances the other: Workers in love look forward to coming to work and enjoying the day; the fact that they are also productive employees benefits the company as well as demonstrates to the lovers that his or her partner is someone to be proud of, someone who takes work seriously and does a thorough job.

Epilogue

The workplace remains a dominant force in our lives. It controls where we live, what time we sleep, and what time we eat. It also impacts our relationships. Some of our richest friendships begin in the workplace. Sometimes these become love relationships that continue long after the building is closed.

Corporate America has moved out of the business of trying to monitor and control the love lives of their employees. With the exception of reporting relationships, employees are trusted to do their jobs and play on their own time. For employees, that means meeting and mating at and through their jobs, absolved of the old guilt (from when dating within the organization was taboo). And they have sex in the office—in risky trysts on the premises, dreamily communicating via their computers, and, often, in their heads. Our Internet survey revealed that almost half of the 774 respondents fantasized about having an emotional or sexual relationship with someone at work. One-fourth of the respondents reported that they had both been in love with and had sex with someone they had met at the office. Some extended their relationships into continued love affairs, living together and marrying.

Our interviews revealed the range of human emotions and experience on the job: from the anguish of sexual harassment and heartbreak when a relationship did not take wing to the adventure, exhilaration, and fulfillment of a lasting love. Some continued in business together, creating their own mom-and-pop businesses; others continued to succeed at the same institution as partners who meet each other for lunch. Most found the workplace as a context for relationships that gave meaning to their lives. For those who seek love from 9 to 5, our respondents taught us that it is but a blink of the eye away—in an open door, a hello, or a smile. . . .

Appendix A

Office Romance Survey

It is not unusual for people to enjoy the people with whom they work; sometimes these relationships become emotional and intimate. This survey is designed to identify your relationship experiences at the office/job/workplace. Completing this survey is completely voluntary and no compensation is provided for your participation. Should you be willing to participate, you may elect to skip questions and select only those to which you feel comfortable responding. Your responses are confidential and anonymous. There is no "capturing of your email or IP address" when you submit this questionnaire. In addition, no identifying code will be attached to any response. Finally, this questionnaire is to be completed by individuals age 18 and above only. If you are 17 and below, you have received this questionnaire in error, so please disregard it.

1. Sex: ( ) Male
   ( ) Female
2. Regarding religion, you are:
   ( ) Atheist
   ( ) Buddhist
   ( ) Christian
   ( ) Hindu
   ( ) Islamic
   ( ) Jewish
   ( ) Other
   ( ) Spiritual, but do not identify with a religion
3. On your last birthday, how old were you? ____
4. What is your highest level of completed education?
   ( ) less than high school diploma/GRE
   ( ) completed/passed GRE

( ) graduated high school
( ) now in college/some college
( ) graduated college
( ) in graduate school/some graduate school
( ) graduated with an MA
( ) graduated with a Ph.D.

5. If currently in college, what year are you?
( ) freshmen ( ) sophomore ( ) junior ( ) senior
( ) not currently in college

6. Which of the following best describes your current relationship situation?
( ) not dating or involved with anyone
( ) casually seeing different people
( ) emotionally involved with the one person I am dating
( ) living together
( ) engaged
( ) married
( ) divorced/separated
( ) other _____

7. What type of place do you work or did you work?
( ) at an office
( ) from my home
( ) travel: do not have an "office"
( ) in a service position: sales, fast food, retail
( ) medical context
( ) academic context
( ) financial context
( ) military
( ) other_____

8. Regarding religion, you are:
( ) very religious
( ) moderately religious
( ) about midway
( ) moderately religious
( ) not religious at all

9. I have a very positive self-concept.

Strongly Agree	Agree	Neither Agree nor Disagree	Disagree	Strongly Disagree
1	2	3	4	5

10. What is the approximate size of the town in which you work?
    ( ) in a small rural area
    ( ) in a moderate city (size = under 50,000)
    ( ) in a moderately large urban area (50,000 to 100,000)
    ( ) in a large urban area (over 100,000)
11. I think of the workplace as a place to meet a mate.

Strongly Agree	Agree	Neither Agree nor Disagree	Disagree	Strongly Disagree
1	2	3	4	5

12. I think of my work as a "job" rather than a "career."

Strongly Agree	Agree	Neither Agree nor Disagree	Disagree	Strongly Disagree
1	2	3	4	5

13. I have been emotionally involved with someone whom I met at work.
    ( ) yes
    ( ) no
14. I have fantasized about having a relationship with a person at work.
    ( ) yes
    ( ) no
15. I have fantasized about having sex with a person at work.
    ( ) yes
    ( ) no
16. I have been sexually involved with a person with whom I worked.
    ( ) yes
    ( ) no
17. The rank of the person I became emotionally involved with at work was (if there has been more than one person, answer in reference to the last person):
    ( ) my boss or someone above me
    ( ) my peer/co-worker
    ( ) someone below me in rank
18. I have lived with someone that I met at work.
    ( ) yes
    ( ) no

19. The rank of the person I became sexually involved with at work was (if there has been more than one person, answer in reference to the last person):
    ( ) my boss or someone above me
    ( ) my peer/co-worker
    ( ) someone below me in rank
20. Has a person at work ever physically touched you in a way that made you uncomfortable?
    ( ) yes
    ( ) no
21. Has a person at work ever said anything sexual to you that made you uncomfortable?
    ( ) yes
    ( ) no
22. Have you ever filed a formal complaint of sexual harassment against someone at work?
    ( ) yes
    ( ) no
23. If you have had an office romance, how did it end? (if there has been more than one person, answer in reference to the last person):
    ( ) we broke up and are no longer friends
    ( ) we broke up and are still friends
    ( ) we are still seeing each other
    ( ) we are living together
    ( ) we are married
24. I have kissed a person at work.
    ( ) yes
    ( ) no
25. I have had oral sex with a person at work.
    ( ) yes
    ( ) no
26. How long did your office romance last?
    ( ) under six months
    ( ) six months to one year
    ( ) one year
    ( ) two years
    ( ) three years
    ( ) four years
    ( ) five years
    ( ) more than five years
    ( ) I have not had an office romance
27. I know _____ people who are or have been involved in a romance with someone they met at work.

( ) none
( ) one
( ) two
( ) three
( ) four
( ) five or more

28. Most of the office romances I know about have had a positive outcome.

Strongly Agree	Agree	Neither Agree nor Disagree	Disagree	Strongly Disagree
1	2	3	4	5

29. I think men exploit women sexually in the workplace.

Strongly Agree	Agree	Neither Agree nor Disagree	Disagree	Strongly Disagree
1	2	3	4	5

30. I was already involved with someone else when I became attracted to someone at work.
    ( ) yes
    ( ) no
    ( ) does not apply
31. I initiated the relationship with the person with whom I became involved at work.
    ( ) yes
    ( ) no
    ( ) not applicable
32. The other person initiated our becoming involved in a relationship at work.
    ( ) yes
    ( ) no
    ( ) not applicable
33. I have been involved in _____ office or workplace romances.
    ( ) none
    ( ) one
    ( ) two
    ( ) three

( ) four
( ) five or more
34. The result of my becoming involved with someone at work was positive
    (if there has been more than one, answer in reference to the most recent
    one).

Strongly Agree	Agree	Neither Agree nor Disagree	Disagree	Strongly Disagree
1	2	3	4	5

Please explain: _____

35. Becoming involved in an office romance was associated with my
    increased productivity at work.

Strongly Agree	Agree	Neither Agree nor Disagree	Disagree	Strongly Disagree
1	2	3	4	5

Please explain: _____

36. Compared with other relationships, the office romance was more diffi-
    cult to end.
    ( ) yes
    ( ) no
    ( ) not applicable

37. I look back on my office romance with regret.

Strongly Agree	Agree	Neither Agree nor Disagree	Disagree	Strongly Disagree	N/A
1	2	3	4	5	6

38. The person I became involved with at the office was:
    ( ) single (or divorced) and available
    ( ) living with someone else at the time
    ( ) emotionally involved with someone else
    ( ) married but separated, not yet divorced
    ( ) married (not separated)
    ( ) not applicable

39. When I became involved with someone at work, I was:
    ( ) single (or divorced) and available
    ( ) living with someone else at the time
    ( ) emotionally involved with someone else
    ( ) married but separated, not yet divorced
    ( ) married (not separated)
    ( ) not applicable
40. The result of my becoming involved with someone at work was negative (if more than one, answer in reference to the most recent one).

Strongly Agree	Agree	Neither Agree nor Disagree	Disagree	Strongly Disagree	N/A
1	2	3	4	5	6

41. I recommend being open to an office romance.

Strongly Agree	Agree	Neither Agree nor Disagree	Disagree	Strongly Disagree
1	2	3	4	5

42. I recommend avoiding an office romance.

Strongly Agree	Agree	Neither Agree nor Disagree	Disagree	Strongly Disagree
1	2	3	4	5

43. I ended up losing the job where I became involved in an office romance (if there has been more than one office romance, answer in reference to the most recent one).
    ( ) yes
    ( ) no
    ( ) not applicable
44. The office romance had a positive influence on my work performance (if more has been more than one office romance, answer in reference to the most recent one).

( ) yes
( ) no
( ) not applicable
45. I work online and became involved with someone I met online during the course of my work.
( ) yes
( ) no
( ) not applicable
46. The result of this online romance was that we:
( ) broke up
( ) are still involved
( ) not applicable
47. I would discourage someone who was about to become involved in an office romance.

Strongly Agree	Agree	Neither Agree nor Disagree	Disagree	Strongly Disagree
1	2	3	4	5

48. I told at least one other person of my office romance.
( ) yes
( ) no
( ) not applicable
49. Other people at work or on the job knew that I was involved in an office romance.
( ) yes
( ) no
( ) maybe
( ) do not know
50. Do you take a shower before work?
( ) yes
( ) no
( ) sometimes
51. Do you wear fresh clothes to work?
( ) yes
( ) no
( ) sometimes
52. How many cups of coffee will you drink before or during your day at the place where you work?
( ) zero
( ) one
( ) two

( ) three
( ) four
( ) five
( ) six or more

53. Have you seen one or more episodes of the television comedy *The Office*?
( ) yes
( ) no

54. Have you seen one or more episodes of the television drama *Mad Men*?
( ) yes
( ) no

THANK YOU FOR COMPLETING THIS SURVEY!

Appendix B

Interview Questions

These questions are designed to elicit your experience and knowledge of office romances. Your answers will be held in confidence. If portions of your answers are used in the book, your data will be disguised in terms of demographic information, and elements of your story will be altered so that they will not reveal your identity. First, some basic information:

Age ____   Type of place where you worked most recently (retail, medical, academic, etc.) _____

Sex ____   Relationship status (single, married, etc.) _____

Education _____

1. Feelings at Work: To what degree have you ever developed emotional feelings for a co-worker? To what degree did you let the person know of these feelings? To what degree did the person reciprocate these feelings?
2. Dating: Have you dated someone whom you met at work? For how long? If it ended, how, why, and by whom? What was your feeling in retrospect about having dated this person? How did dating change your feeling about your work/job?
3. What was the status of this person in reference to you ... your boss, your co-worker, a person you supervised?
4. What was your goal in dating this person ... a good time, sex, love, a mate?
5. How open were you to other co-workers about dating this person?
6. Aside from dating a co-worker, have you dated someone whom you met through work at a conference, or through a client, or because of some aspect of your job?
7. To what degree do you view yourself as a flirt at work?
8. To what degree have you fantasized about emotional or sexual involvement with a person at work? Do you regret not acting on your fantasy?

9. Have you gone out on a date with a boss?
10. Were you ever involved in an affair with a boss?
11. Have you gone out with a subordinate?
12. Did the relationship with the boss or subordinate include sex?
13. Are you aware of a sexual harassment lawsuit against someone at your place of work?
14. Have you considered marrying someone you met at the office? ?
15. How was the romance with someone at work different from your having met the partner elsewhere?
16. To what degree is your work a "career" versus a "job"?
17. What are your thoughts on keeping an office romance a secret?
18. How many people do you know who met at work and subsequently married? Can you tell their story (anonymously)? If one is your friend, might I speak with him or her?
19. What would you advise someone who has an interest in dating someone at work?
20. If you are single, to what degree do you regard the job as a place to meet a potential spouse?
21. How does the workplace as a place to meet people compare to other alternatives?
22. What is the official policy of your place of work toward emotional/sexual relationship among co-workers? Have you read it or heard it discussed— do you think it's important to be aware of it? Do you think your employer is relaxed or critical about love relationships that may develop among employees?
23. When people who are employed in the same place marry, should they continue to work in the same place? How are married couples to work with?
24. Do you consider yourself ambitious in terms of your career? How has being focused on your career affected your having an office romance, or how might it in the future?
25. What are your feelings about looking for a partner via the office, Internet, church, friends, etc.?
26. If you married a person you met at work, how did your being married affect your job? How did it affect the relationship with your partner?
27. To what degree have you felt sexually harassed by a superior at work? To what degree have you felt that women at the office were given special favors because they were having sex with the boss?
28. Do you work at home on a computer? To what degree have you "emotionally connected" with someone you were "working with" online? Did the relationship escalate? What happened?
29. What was not asked that you have experienced about office romances? What do people thinking about an office romance need to know?

Notes

Chapter 1: Who's Playing at Work?

1. *Statistical Abstract of the United States: 2010*, 129th ed. (Washington, D.C.: U.S. Government Printing Office), Table 57.

2. Ibid.

3. R. E. Quinn, "Management of Romantic Relationships in Organizations," *Administrative Science Quarterly* 22 (1977): 30–45.

4. *Statistical Abstract of the United States: 2010*, 129th ed. (Washington, D.C.: U.S. Government Printing Office), Table 57.

5. Ibid.

6. Y. K. Djama, M. J. Crump, and A. G. Jackson, "Levels and Determinants of Extramarital Sex." Paper presented at Southern Sociological Society, Charlotte, NC (March, 2005).

7. Phil Stott, "No Recession for Workplace Romance," Vault.Com Office Romance Survey 2010, http://vaultcareers.wordpress.com/2010/02/17/no-recession-for-workplace-romance/ (retrieved February 18, 2010).

8. Interview with Dr. Marie G. McIntyre, January 12, 2010.

Chapter 2: Eleven Types of Office Loves

1. O. Fred Donaldson, *Playing by Heart: The Vision and Practice of Belonging* (Deerfield Beach, FL: Health Communications, 1993).

2. C. J. Anderson, and C. Fisher, "Male-Female Relationships in the Workplace: Perceived Motivations in Office Romance," *Sex Roles* 25 (1991): 163–180.

3. "Forty Percent of Workers Have Dated a Co-Worker, Finds Annual CareerBuilder.com Valentine's Day Survey," CareerBuilder.com, http://www.careerbuilder.com/share/aboutus/pressreleasesdetail.aspx?id=pr553&sd=2%2f9%2f2010&ed=12%2f31%2f2010&siteid=cbpr&sc_cmp1=cb_pr553_&

cbRecursionCnt=1&cbsid=9354b8fc6d164b7cad8a6ed186882567-319524618
-VM-4 (retrieved February 15, 2010).

4. Phil Stott, "No Recession for Workplace Romance," Vault.Com Office Romance Survey 2010, http://vaultcareers.wordpress.com/2010/02/17/no-recession-for-workplace-romance/(retrieved February 18, 2010).

5. Ibid.

6. R. E. Quinn, "Management of Romantic Relationships in Organizations," *Administrative Science Quarterly* 22 (1977): 30–45.

7. CareerBuilder.com.

Chapter 3: The Upside of Office Romances

1. C. A. Pierce, "Factors Associated with Participating in a Romantic Relationship in a Work Environment." *Journal of Applied Social Psychology*, 28 (1998): 1712–1730.

2. J. Lever, G. Zellman, and S. J. Hirschfeld, "Office Romance: Are the Rules Changing?" *Across the Board* (March/April, 2006), pp. 33–41.

Chapter 4: Virtual Office: Love Online

1. J. J. Cameron and M. Ross, "In Times of Uncertainty: Predicting the Survival of Long-Distance Relationships," *Journal of Social Psychology* 147 (2007): 581–604.

2. G. T. Guldner, *Long Distance Relationships: The Complete Guide* (Corona, California: JF Milne Publications, 2003).

3. D. Knox, M. Zusman, V. Daniels, and A. Brantley, "Absence Makes the Heart Grow Fonder? Long-Distance Dating Relationships Among College Students," *College Student Journal* 36 (2002): 365–367.

4. J. Lydon, T. Pierce, and S. O'Regan, "Coping with Moral Commitment to Long-Distance Dating Relationships," *Journal of Personality and Social Psychology* 73 (1997): 104–113.

5. K. C. Maguire, "Will It Ever End?: A (Re)examination of Uncertainty in College Student Long-Distance Dating Relationships," *Communication Quarterly* 55 (2007): 415–432.

6. D. Gardiner, "A Sniff of Your Sweetie," *Psychology Today* 38 (2005): 31–32.

Chapter 5: Office Romance Etiquette

1. Interview with Janie Chang, November 7, 2009.

2. J. Lever, G. Zellman, and S. J. Hirschfeld, "Romance in the Office," *The Conference Board Review Magazine* (March/April, 2006).

3. J. L. Berdahl, J. L. Rotman, and K. Aquino, "Sexual Behavior at Work: Fun or Folly?," *Journal of Applied Psychology* 94 (2009): 9002–9010.

4. Interview with Dr. Marie G. McIntyre, January 12, 2010.

5. "'Mrs. Robinson Scandal' Ousts Irish Leader," CBS News–World, January 11, 2010.

Chapter 6: Dating Up and Down the Ranks

1. "Forty Percent of Workers Have Dated a Co-Worker, Finds Annual CareerBuilder.com Valentine's Day Survey," CareerBuilder.com, http://www .careerbuilder.com/share/aboutus/pressreleasesdetail.aspx?id=pr553& sd=2%2f9%2f2010&ed=12%2f31%2f2010&siteid=cbpr&sc_cmp1=cb_pr553 _&cbRecursionCnt=1&cbsid=9354b8fc6d164b7cad8a6ed186882567-319524618 -VM-4 (retrieved February 15, 2010).

2. C. J. Anderson and C. Fisher, "Male-Female Relationships in the Workplace: Perceived Motivations in Office Romance," *Sex Roles* 25 (1991): 163–180.

3. M. Roehm and M. K. Brady, "Consumer Responses to Performance Failures by High-Equity Brands," *Journal of Consumer Research* 34 (2007): 537–545.

4. Used by permission of Jeffrey M. Tanenbaum, Partner, Nixon Peabody LLP, One Embarcadero Center, 18th Floor, San Francisco, CA 94111-3600.

5. "Pregnant Troops Leave the War; Central Command Not Counting," *The Washington Times* online, June 15, 2004.

6. "Kate Wiltrout, "Destroyer CO, Master Chief Removed over Fraternization Cases," The *Virginian-Pilot*, December 4, 2009, www.freerepublic.com/ focus/news/2400.

7. Teri Weaver, "U.S. Personnel in Iraq Could Face Court-Martial for Getting Pregnant," *Stars & Stripes*, December 19, 2009.

8. G. E. Jones, "Hierarchical Workplace Romance: An Experimental Examination of Team Member Perceptions," *Journal of Organizational Behavior* 20 (1999): 1057–1072.

9. L. Hochwald, "Vows—Gita Pullapilly and Aron Gaudet," *The New York Times*, November 1, 2009, p. 14L (late edition).

10. March 9, 2010 Interview with Jeff Tanenbaum, Chair of Nixon Peabody's Labor & Employment Group, Nixon Peabody LLP, One Embarcadero Center, 18th Floor, San Francisco, CA 94111.

Chapter 7: What He Is Thinking

1. J. Colapinto, *As Nature Made Him: The Boy Who Was Raised as a Girl* (New York: Harper Collins, 2000).

2. A. D. Neely, D. Knox, and M. Zusman, "College Student Beliefs About Women: Some Gender Differences," *College Student Journal* 39 (2005): 769–774.

3. *Statistical Abstract of the United States: 2010*, 129th ed. (Washington, D.C.: U.S. Government Printing Office), Table 57.

4. R. Thornhill and C. T. Palmer, *A Natural History of Rape: Biological Bases of Sexual Coercion* (Cambridge, MA: MIT Press, 2000).

5. C. J. Fisher and C. Fisher, "Male-Female Relationships in the Workplace: Perceived Motivations in Office Romance," *Sex Roles* 25 (1991): 163–180.

6. M. W. Wiederman, "Extramarital Sex: Prevalence and Correlates in a National Survey," *The Journal of Sex Research* 34 (1997): 167–174.

7. A. R. McAlister, N. Pachana, and C. J. Jackson, "Predictors of Young Dating Adult's Inclination to Engage in Extradyadic Sexual Activities: A Multi-Perspective Study," *British Journal of Psychology* 96 (2005): 331–350.

8. C. J. Fisher and C. Fisher, "Male-Female Relationships in the Workplace: Perceived Motivations in Office Romance," *Sex Roles* 25 (1991): 163–180.

9. Ibid.

10. Ibid.

Chapter 8: What She Is Thinking

1. J. Sparks, *Battle of the Sexes: the Natural History of Sex* (Darby, Pennsylvania: Diane Publishing Co., 2001), p. 40.

2. O. Judson, *Dr. Tatiana's Sex Advice to All Creation* (New York: Holt, 2002), p. 17.

Chapter 9: Men to Avoid at the Office

1. G. Orwell, "Pleasure Spots," in *In Front of Your Nose: The Collected Essays*, (New York: Harcourt Brace Jovanovich, 1945–1950).

2. Inteview with Dr. Agnes Wilkie, January 28, 2010.

3. W. A. Nolen, *Crisis Time!: Love, Marriage and the Male at Midlife* (New York: Dodd Mead, 1984), pp.115–116.

4. A. Young, *The Politician*, (New York: Thomas Dunne Books, 2010).

5. L. K. Stroh, *Trust Rules: How to Tell the Good Guys from the Bad Guys in Work and Life*, (Westport, CT: Praeger, 2007), p. 91.

Chapter 10: Men to Include in your Office Search

1. D. Brian, *The Curies: The Untold Story Behind Their Private and Professional Lives* (Hoboken, New Jersey: Wily, 2005).

2. *Statistical Abstract of the United States: 2010*, 129th ed. (Washington, D.C.: U.S. Government Printing Office), Table 57.

3. Ibid.

4. *Statistical Abstract of the United States: 2010*, 129th ed. (Washington, D.C.: U.S. Government Printing Office), Table 60.

5. M. R. Hill and V. Thomas, "Strategies for Racial Identity Development: Narratives of Black and White Women in Interracial Relationships," *Family Relations* 49 (2000): 193–200.

6. S. O. Gaines, Jr., and J. Leaver, "Interracial Relationships," in *Inappropriate Relationships: The Unconventional, the Disapproved, and the Forbidden*, ed. by R. Goodwin and D. Cramer (Florence, Kentucky: Lawrence Erlbaum, 2002): 65–78.

7. D. A. Kreaer, "Guarded Borders: Adolescent Interracial Romance and Peer Trouble at School," *Social Forces* 87 (2008): 887–910.

8. K. Barnes and J. Patrick, "Examining Age-Congruency and Marital Satisfaction," *The Gerontologist* 44 (2004): 185–187.

9. Pew Forum on Religion Public Life, (2008), "The U.S. Religious Landscape Survey," http://pewresearch.org/pubs/743/united-states-religion.

10. *Statistical Abstract of the United States: 2010*, 129th ed. (Washington, D.C.: U.S. Government Printing Office), Table 44.

11. D. Knox and M. E. Zusman, "Relationship and Sexual Behaviors of a Sample of 1319 University Students," Department of Sociology, East Carolina University, unpublished data.

12. Interview with Leia Cain, January 30, 2010.

Chapter 11: Should you Marry your Office Love?

1. "Forty Percent of Workers Have Dated a Co-Worker, Finds Annual CareerBuilder.com Valentine's Day Survey," CareerBuilder.com, http://www .careerbuilder.com/share/aboutus/pressreleasesdetail.aspx?id=pr553& sd=2%2f9%2f2010&ed=12%2f31%2f2010&siteid=cbpr&sc_cmp1=cb_pr553 _&cbRecursionCnt=1&cbsid=9354b8fc6d164b7cad8a6ed186882567-319524618 -VM-4 (retrieved February 15, 2010).

2. K. K. Assad, M. B. Donnellan, and R. D. Conger, "Optimism: An Enduring Resource for Romantic Relationships," *Journal of Personality and Social Psychology* 93 (2007): 285–296.

3. J. D. Foster, "Incorporating Personality into the Investment Model: Probing Commitment Processes across Individual Differences in Narcissism," *Journal of Social and Personal Relationships* 25 (2008): 211–223.

4. K. S. Gattis, S. Berns, L. E. Simpson and A. Christensen, "Birds of a Feather or Strange Birds? Ties Among Personality Dimensions, Similarity, and Marital Quality," *Journal of Family Psychology* 18 (2004): 564–578.

5. D. K. Snyder and J. M. Regts, "Personality Correlates of Marital Satisfaction: A Comparison of Psychiatric, Maritally Distressed, and Nonclinic Samples," *Journal of Sex and Marital Therapy* 19 (1990): 34–43.

6. Ibid.

7. M. Haring, P. L. Hewitt, and G. L. Flett, "Perfectionism, Coping, and Quality of Relationships," *Journal of Marriage and the Family* 65 (2003): 143–159.

8. Crowell, J., A. D. Treboux, and E. Waters, "Stability of Attachment Representations. The Transition to Marriage," *Developmental Psychology* 38 (2002): 467–479.

9. Huston, T. L., J. P. Caughlin, R. M. Houts, S. E. Smith, and L. J. George, "The Connubial Crucible: Newlywed Years as Predictors of Marital Delight, Distress, and Divorce," *Journal of Personality and Social Psychology* 80 (2001): 237–252.

10. P. R. Amato, A. Booth, D. R. Johnson, and S. F. Rogers, *Alone Together: How Marriage in America Is Changing* (Cambridge, Massachusetts: Harvard University Press, 2007).

11. E. E. Pimentel, "Just How Do I Love Thee? Marital Relations in Urban China," *Marriage and the Family* 62 (2000): 32–47.

12. P. R. Amato, A. Booth, D. R. Johnson, and S. F. Rogers, *Alone Together: How Marriage in America Is Changing* (Cambridge, Massachusetts: Harvard University Press, 2007).

13. J. M. Torpy, C. Lynm, and R. M. Glass, "Intimate partner violence," *Journal of the American Medical Association* 300 (2008): 754–766.

14. D. Knox and M. Zusman, "Become Involved with Someone on the Rebound: How Fast Should You Run?," *College Student Journal* 43 (2009): 99–104.

15. Interview with Dr. Marie G. McIntyre, January 12, 2010.

Chapter 12: Trade Secrets of the Ultimate Office Romance

1. "Forty Percent of Workers Have Dated a Co-Worker, Finds Annual CareerBuilder.com Valentine's Day Survey," CareerBuilder.com, http://www .careerbuilder.com/share/aboutus/pressreleasesdetail.aspx?id=pr481& sd=2/10/2009&ed=12/31/2009&cbRecursionCnt=1&cbsid=2bf18201bff24ed 890476ca06e69c917-316363568-KA-5&ns_siteid=ns_us_g_careerbuilder.com _200_ (retrieved January 9, 2010).

2. Ibid.

3. Ibid.

4. J. Merrill and D. Knox, *When I Fall in Love Again: A New Study on Finding and Keeping the Love of Your Life* (Santa Barbara, CA: ABC-CLIO, 2010). Chapter 1, Table 1.

5. Ibid., Chapter 1, Table 2.

6. Ibid., Chapter 1, Table 1.

7. Ibid.

8. Ibid.

9. CareerBuilder.com.

10. Ibid.

11. Ibid.

12. D. Knox, D., and M. Zusman, "Relationship and Sexual Behaviors of a Sample of 1319 University Students," Department of Sociology, East Carolina University, Greenville, NC. (2009), unpublished data.

13. K. Vail-Smith, L. MacKenzie, and D. Knox, "Illusion of Safety in Monogamous Relationships," *American Journal of Health Behavior* 34 (2010): 12–20.

14. Interview with Dr. Lois Frankel, January 7, 2010.

Chapter 13: When the office Romance Becomes Sexual

1. "Forty Percent of Workers Have Dated a Co-Worker, Finds Annual CareerBuilder.com Valentine's Day Survey," CareerBuilder.com, http://www .careerbuilder.com/share/aboutus/pressreleasesdetail.aspx?id=pr553& sd=2%2f9%2f2010&ed=12%2f31%2f2010&siteid=cbpr&sc_cmp1=cb_pr553_&

cbRecursionCnt=1&cbsid=9354b8fc6d164b7cad8a6ed186882567-319524618
-VM-4 (retrieved February 15, 2010).

2. Maryanne Vandervelde, *The Changing Life of a Corporate Wife* (New York: Mecox Publishing, 1979).

3. Interview with Brigadier General Walter E. Lippincott (retired) of the National Guard, January 10, 2010.

4. D. Knox and B. Brigman, "University Students Reaction to Intercourse," *College Student Journal* 30 (1996): 547–548.

5. S. S. Rostosky, D. Welsh, M. C. Kawaguchi, and R. V. Galliher, "Commitment and Sexual Behaviors in Adolescent Dating Relationships," in *Handbook of Interpersonal Commitment and Relationship Stability*, ed. by J. M. Adams and W. H. Jones (New York: Academic/Plenum Publishers, 1999), pp. 223–228.

6. D. Knox, L. Sturdivant, and M. E. Zusman, "College Student Attitudes Toward Sexual Intimacy," *College Student Journal* 35 (2001): 241–243.

7. D. Knox, L. Sturdivant, and M. E. Zusman, "College Student Attitudes Toward Sexual Intimacy," *College Student Journal* 35 (2001): 241–243.

8. Interview conducted by Adam Bryant, *New York Times* Business Section, July 26, 2009.

9. R. T. Michael, J. H. Gagnon, E. O. Laumann, and G. Kolata, *Sex in America* (Boston: Little, Brown, 1994).

10. "Pregnant G.I's Could be Punished," Associated Press, December 19, 2009.

Chapter 15: Being in Business/Working Together

1. *Statistical Abstract of the United States: 2010*, 129th ed. (Washington, D.C.: U.S. Government Printing Office), Table 687.

2. R. Morin and D. Cohn, "Women Call All the Shots at Home; Public Mixed on Gender Roles in Job, Gender and Power," Pew Research Center, September 25, 2008.

3. R. Schoen, N. M. Astone, K. Rothert, N. J. Standish, and Y. J. Kim, "Women's Employment, Marital Happiness, and Divorce" *Social Forces* 81 (2002): 643–62.

4. J. R. Gordon and K. S. Whelan-Berry, "Contributions to Family and Household Activities by the Husbands of Midlife Professional Women," *Journal of Family Studies* 26 (2005): 899–923.

5. S. N. Rodriguez, G. Hildreth, and J. Mancuso, "The Dynamics of Families in Business: How Therapists Can Help in Ways Consultants Don't," *Contemporary Family Therapy: An International Journal* 21 (1999): 453–472.

6. S. Nelton, *In Love and in Business: How Entrepreneurial Couples Are Changing the Roles of Business and Marriage* (New York: John Wiley, 1986).

7. *The Complete Romances of Chretien de Troyes*, trans. David Staines (Bloomington, Indiana: Indiana University Press, 1990), p. 31.

8. Ibid., p. 61.

9. Interview with John Wertime, December 11, 2009.

10. Michael T. Kaufman, "William H. Whyte, 'Organization Man,' Author and Urbanologist, Is Dead at 81, *New York Times*, January 13, 1999.

11. Interview with Leigh Cousins, November 18, 2009.

12. E. Coleman, *Four-Season Harvest by Eliot Coleman* (White River Junction, VT: Chelsea Green Press, 1999), p. 13

13. Henry David Thoreau, *Journal 23*, January 1841. *The Writings of Henry David Thoreau*. Journal, Vol 1., 1837–1846 (Boston: Houghton Mifflin, The Riverside Press, 1906), chapter V, 1841, p. 174.

14. Interview with Lisa A. Maniero, December 28, 2009.

15. Londa Schiebinger, A. D. Henderson, and S. K. Gilmartin, *Dual-Career Academic Couples: What Universities Need to Know* (Stanford, California: Board of Trustees of the Leland Stanford Junior University, 2008), http://www.stanford.edu/group/gender/ResearchPrograms/DualCareer/index.html.

16. Interview with Leigh Cousins, January 7, 2010.

17. George Robert Bach, *The Intimate Enemy: How to Fight Fair in Love and Marriage* (New York: Morrow, 1999).

18. J. Huizinga, *Homo Ludens* (Boston, MA: Beacon Press, 1950), p. 211.

19. K. Vail-Smith, D. Knox, and M. Zusman, "The Lonely College Male," *International Journal of Men's Health*, 6 (2007): 273–279.

20. G. L. Grief, "Male Friendships: Implications from Research on Family Therapy," *Family Therapy*, 33 (2006): 1–15.

21. D. Maume, "Gender Differences in Taking Vacation Time," *Work and Occupations*, 33 (2006): 161–190.

22. "The Colin McEnroe Show," National Public Radio, Dec 15, 2009.

23. Margaret Mead, *Blackberry Winter: My Earliest Years* (NY: William and Morrow Company, 1972), p. 181.

Chapter 16: If the Office Romance Ends

1. M. Shikibu, *The Tale of Genji*, ed. By Edward G. Seidensticker, vol. 2 (New York: Alfred A. Knopf, 1976), p. 2.

2. T. Tetlie, N. Eik-Nes, T. Pamstierma, P. Callaghan, and J. A. Nottestad, "The Effect of Exercise on Psychological and Physical Health Outcomes: Preliminary Results from a Norwegian Forensic Hospital," *Journal of Psychosocial Nursing and Mental Health Services* 46 (2008): 38–44.

3. For more information on a government-funded study on veterans who take yoga, see http://clinicaltrials.gov/ct2/show/NCT00962403?term=khalsa&rank=1.

4. E. Kubler-Ross, *On Death and Dying* (New York: Collier Books of Macmillan, 1969).

5. F. Bacon, "Of Revenge," in *The Oxford Book of Essays*, ed. by John Gross (New York: Oxford University Press, 1991), p. 4.

Chapter 17: Office Romance Policies and Sexual Harassment

1. Phil Stott, "No Recession for Workplace Romance," Vault.Com Office Romance Survey, 2010, http://vaultcareers.wordpress.com/2010/02/17/no-recession-for-workplace-romance/ (retrieved February 18, 2010).

2. "Cupid Finds Work as Office Romance no Longer Taboo—Changing Attitudes, Long Hours Open Door to Love," *USA Today* (2003), Money section, p. 1b.

3. B. Gregg, (2005), "Restrictions on Workplace Romance and Consensual Relationship Policies," Boardman Law Firm of Madison, Wisconsin, http://www.boardmanlawfirm.com/perspectives_articles/workplace_romance.html (retrieved November 17, 2009).

4. Ibid.

5. W. L. O'Neill, "Sex Scandals in the Gender-Integrated Military," *Gender Issues* 16 (1998): 64–47.

6. B. L. Roach, "Walking the Diversity Compliance Tightrope: Maintaining the Balance between Enforcement and Equity," *Forum on Public Policy* (2006).

7. Ibid.

8. M. Parks, "Workplace Romance Poll Findings," *Society for Human Resource Management (SHRM) Report* (Alexandria, VA: 2006).

9. Ibid.

10. B. E. Schneider, "Myth and Reality for Heterosexual and Lesbian Women Workers," *Sociological Perspectives* 27 (1984): 443–464.

11. C. Uggen, and A. Blackstone, "Sexual Harassment as a Gendered Expression of Power," *American Sociological Review* 69 (2005): 64–92.

12. J. A. Richman, K. M. Rospenda, S. J. Nawyn, J. A. Flaherty, M. Fendrich, and M. L. Drum, et al., "Sexual Harassment and Generalized Workplace Abuse," in *Speaking of Sexuality*, ed. by J. K. Davidson, Sr. and N. B. Moore (Los Angeles, CA: Roxbury Publishing Co, 2001).

13. C. Avina and W. O'Donohue, "Sexual Harassment and PTSD: Is Sexual Harassment Diagnosable Trauma?," *Journal of Traumatic Stress* 15 (2002): 69–75.

14. A. E. Street, J. Stafford, C. M. Mahan and A. Hendricks, "Sexual Harassment and Assault Experienced by Reservists during Military Service: Prevalence and Health Correlates," *Journal of Rehabilitation Research & Development* 45 (2008): 409–420.

15. Harris Interactive & Witeck-Combs, *Sexual Harassment Among Gay and Lesbian Employees,* Out and Equal Workplace Conference, Orlando, Florida, September, 2002.

16. T. P. Sbraga and W. O'Donohue, "Sexual Harassment," *Annual Review of Sex Research* 11 (2000): 258–285.

17. E. O'Hare and W. O'Donohue, "Sexual Harassment: Identifying Risk Factors," *Archives of Sexual Behavior* 27 (1998): 561–579.

18. N. Gibbs, "The War Within," *Time*, March 8, 2010, p. 60.

19. K. L. Wuensch, M. W. Campbell, K. C. Kesler, and C. H. Moore, "Racial Bias in Decisions Made by Mock Jurors Evaluating a Case of Sexual Harassment," *The Journal of Social Psychology* 142 (2002): 587–600.

20. J. Matchen and E. DeSouza, "The Sexual Harassment of Faculty Members by Students," *Sex Roles* 42 (2000): 295–306.

21. R. Eisenman, "The Fair and Unfair Sexual Harassment Charge," *Journal of Evolutionary Psychology* 34 (2000): 34–40.

22. S. Fineran, "Sexual Harassment between Same-Sex Peers: Intersection of Mental Health, Homophobia, and Sexual Violence in Schools," *Social Work* 47 (2000): 65–74.

23. C. Avina and W. O'Donohue, "Sexual Harassment and PTSD: Is Sexual Harassment Diagnosable Trauma?," *Journal of Traumatic Stress* 15 (2002): 69–75.

24. B. S. Dansky and D. G. Kilpatrick, "Effects of Sexual Harassment," in *Sexual Harassment: Theory, Research, and Treatment*, ed by W. O'Donohue (Needham Heights, MA: Allyn & Bacon, 1997), pp. 152–174.

25. Ibid.

26. Sexual Harassment Chargers: EEOC & FEPAs Combined: 1997–2008, http://www.eeoc.gov/eeoc/statistics/enforcement/sexual_harassment.cfm.

27. T. P. Sbraga and W. O'Donohue, "Sexual Harassment," *Annual Review of Sex Research* 11 (2000): 258–285.

28. J. L. Pershing, "Why Women Don't Report Sexual Harassment: A Case Study of An Elite Military Institution," *Gender Issues* 21 (2003): 3–30.

29. J. Gross, "Ideas and Trends: Now Look Who's Taunting. Now Look Who's Suing? *New York Times*, December 10, 2009, p. 41.

30. Interview with Dr. Marie G. McIntyre, January 12, 2010.

31. *State of Nevada Employee Handbook*, Department of Personnel, Blasdel Building, 209 East Musser Street, Room 101, Carson City, Nevada 89701-4204, July, 2009, http://www.dop.nv.gov.

32. *Tenge vs. Phillips Modern Ag. Co.*, U.S. Court of Appeals, Eighth Circuit (2006).

Index

About the Authors

JANE MERRILL has written eight books and more than 50 relationship articles for magazines such as *Redbook*, *Vogue*, and *Cosmopolitan*. She is the co-author (with David Knox) of *When I Fall in Love Again: A New Study on Finding and Keeping the Love of Your Life* (Praeger).

DAVID KNOX, Ph.D., is professor of sociology at East Carolina University, Greenville, NC, where he teaches courses on courtship and marriage, marriage and family, and human sexuality. He is the author or coauthor of 90 professional articles and 10 books, including *Choices in Relationships: An Introduction to Marriage and Family*, 10th edition, and *Choices in Sexuality*.